365 Easy
One-Dish Meals

Other books in this series are:

365 WAYS TO COOK CHICKEN
365 WAYS TO COOK PASTA
365 QUICK & EASY MICROWAVE RECIPES
365 GREAT BARBECUE & GRILLING RECIPES
365 EASY LOW-CALORIE RECIPES

365 Easy
One-Dish Meals

Natalie Haughton

A JOHN BOSWELL ASSOCIATES BOOK

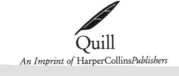

Quill
An Imprint of HarperCollins*Publishers*

HarperCollins books may be purchased
for educational, business, or sales
promotional use. For information please
write: Special Markets Department,
HarperCollins Publishers Inc.,
10 East 53rd Street, New York, NY 10022.

First Quill edition published 2004.

Design: Nigel Rollings
Index: Maro Riofrancos

Library of Congress Cataloging-in-Publication Data is available.
ISBN 0-06-057888-2

04 05 06 07 08 RRD 10 9 8 7 6 5 4 3 2 1

Acknowledgments

Special thanks to my husband, Fred, and children, Alexis and Grant, for coping with me during the recipe development and testing frenzies. Their untiring love, encouragement, and devotion as well as taste-testing help and input were invaluable and greatly appreciated. Thanks, too, to my parents and friends for sharing favorite recipes as well as their enthusiasm for this project; and to Patti Gray, for her generous support (she kept me laughing) and help with recipe development and testing.

Contents

Introduction

While the concept of one-dish meals has been around for a long time, it's still a great way to create a meal, and more appropriate today than ever before.

Why? Because one-dish meals offer cooks an easy solution to preparing great-tasting, nutritious, all-occasion, kind-to-the-budget meals with minimum cleanup. The basic premise is simple—some type of protein, starch (such as rice, pasta, or potatoes), and vegetables or fruits are combined in a single utensil; or if you prefer, you can combine two of the elements, such as protein and vegetables, and serve over a starch of your choice. The aim is to streamline cooking chores and utensils as much as possible and to make cooking and eating, after work or with a hectic family, as enjoyable as possible.

The one-dish concept couldn't be more in step with today's fast-paced lifestyle. In most cases, the recipes in this volume require only the addition of a simple salad or bread to make a complete meal.

One-dish meals offer cooks a wide range of options. You can whip them up in a variety of utensils, or pieces of equipment, ranging from a skillet to a wok to a casserole to a Dutch oven or even a salad bowl to a slow crockery-cooker or a pressure cooker to a microwave oven and much more.

Another big bonus—the cleanup patrol will definitely be singing the cook's praises, since there is only one pot to wash.

Some of the single-dish ideas that follow can be prepared in advance and refrigerated, others can be cooked ahead and reheated or even frozen. Many fill the needs of busy families whose members dine on different schedules. In most cases, you can simply refrigerate and reheat the leftovers as needed, without significant loss of quality. Still others are great potluck offerings.

With more than 50 percent of women working outside the home these days, there just isn't time for lengthy, complicated cooking. One-dish meals are right in tune with the trend back to simpler, homey fare. Whether for daily suppers or company meals, concentrating on a single terrific entrée for the centerpiece of the meal is smart menu planning.

As the busy working mother of two children, I find it easier to put a one-pot dinner on the table than to stop for fast food or serve frozen prepared dinners. It's certainly more nutritious and economical, because I have control over what goes into the dish.

One-pot cooking has been a way of life for our family for the past few years. With time at a premium, it offers flexibility and versatility in turning out tasty, appealing foods with minimal effort. Skillet meals as well as salads, soups (especially the quick ones), and pasta dishes rank high among my family's list of favorites, and many of my tried-and-true recipes can be found within these pages.

One-dish meals can range from hearty and healthy to quick and slow-cooking. You can turn out meals in minutes with a wok or microwave, or bake them lazily in a Dutch oven for several hours. Or you can opt to make a jiffy stove-top skillet meal (by far the largest chapter in this volume because so many of the recipes are energy-saving, quick, and easy) or a stove-top-to-oven casserole or a simple baked casserole, where everything is simply tossed in a single dish. Other options include sandwiches and pizzas prepared in a single pan, as well as salads relying on a single large bowl. Once you get the knack of one-pot meal cooking, it'll transform your cooking style forever.

While fresh foods are preferable and are emphasized in numerous recipes, it is a fact that packaged, frozen, and canned items are extremely convenient. And for emergencies they can be stocked well in advance. I've taken that into account and have designed a generous sprinkling of shortcut recipes—the reach and cook kind. These successfully utilize some of the vast array of convenience products available today, like packaged rice mixes, spaghetti sauce mix, canned soups, canned broths, quick-cooking brown and white rice, etc., which continue to proliferate on supermarket shelves. Although I don't advocate reliance on convenience foods everyday, there are times in a pinch when they come in handy. But heed this word of warning: Be cautious when using today's convenience or processed food products, because many of them contain substantial amounts of sodium. Go easy on the salt in recipes or consider buying reduced-sodium alternatives of products such as soy sauce, chicken broth, soup mixes, and the like.

Half the battle in whipping up one-dish creations efficiently and pleasantly is having the proper utensils on hand. If you plan to make a stove-top-to-oven skillet or casserole, be sure you have a flameproof utensil in your equipment repertoire. Metal or glass skillets with ovenproof handles are available, as are casserole dishes that are at home both on the stove or in the oven.

Likewise, if you're planning to make a pot of soup, be sure that you have a stockpot, Dutch oven, or soup kettle with a nonreactive surface available, particularly if the recipe contains wine, tomatoes, or any acidic foods. Nonreactive means no iron or unclad aluminum.

And if you're planning to invest in some pots, pans, or casseroles to use for one-dish meals, check out the quality, construction, design, and versatility prior to buying. Although it may seem expensive at the time of purchase, it's wise to purchase good-quality cookware, because you'll reap the benefits of its durability and reliability for many years.

Select pots and pans that suit your family size and cooking style and shy away from buying pan sets, which often contain one or two utensils you'll never use. Remember that no one metal is ideal for all cooking purposes.

Copper is an excellent heat conductor, but it will tarnish, it is difficult to keep clean, and the tin lining, which is subject to wear and must be replaced from time to time, will melt if it exceeds 410 degrees. Aluminum is strong and lightweight, and it conducts heat well, but its main drawback is its susceptibility to reaction with acidic foods. Pots that bond the aluminum with other materials, such as Calphalon, overcome this problem. Stainless steel is extremely durable, easy to clean, the least reactive and most practical cooking surface, but its major drawback is its poor heat conductivity as well as its tendency to burn the food in spots. Cast iron cookware, though not a particularly good conductor of heat, maintains heat because of the pot's heavy weight. It is durable and versatile, but is not appropriate for cooking dishes containing wine or acidic foods. Often it lends a metallic taste to foods, and it tends to rust. Another possibility is porcelain-coated cast iron, such as Le Creuset, which is easier to clean, has a nonreactive surface, and is pretty. But such pots are very heavy, expensive, and can chip and crack. All-Clad combines the qualities of aluminum with those of stainless steel for even heating. Anodized aluminum is a good choice for stockpots and saucepans. Before you buy, look around and gather information. I've found it most successful to mix and match cookware styles, types, and materials so I have plenty of options from which to choose on a moment's notice.

From my perspective, a 5- to 6-quart nonreactive Dutch oven that goes from stove-top to oven is one of the best investments you can make if you're planning to cook a lot of one-dish meals. It can double as a soup pot and is wonderful for making chilies, stews, chicken dishes, and stove-top meals.

But I'm also fond of my 10- and 12-inch covered skillets, my 3- and 4-quart saucepans and my professional weight carbon steel wok. Another utensil I've found handy is a round 9-inch covered glass (actually a glasslike, high-temperature ceramic called Pyroceram, which is marketed under the Visions brand label) chicken fryer, which looks like a skillet and measures 9 inches in diameter and is 3 inches deep. It doubles as a microwave cooking utensil as well. And, of course, the myriad sizes and shapes of casseroles and baking dishes are all very useful as well. I would also have a tough time getting along without my 11x7, or 9x13-inch heatproof glass baking dishes, my salad bowls, 10x15-inch jelly-roll pan, pizza pans, and springform pans as well. It's amazing how often these utensils are pressed into service at my house.

Because of the popularity and flexibility of one-pot cooking, the 365 recipes that follow should appeal to a wide variety of cooks and tastes. Some dishes are old-fashioned classics, others are modern and up-scale; still others are fast and easy, and even elegant. All are designed to put a meal on the table with minimal effort and muss and fuss.

If you are one of today's busy cooks, we think you'll agree one-dish meals really are a boon once you try them. You'll have to look long and hard to find a better way to easily prepare a meal.

And now for some wonderful eating! Cheers!

Chapter 1

Dutch Oven: The Stew Pot

Dutch ovens are large pans, generally ranging from 4- to 14-quart capacities, with ear handles and lids. They are invaluable for cooking stews, chiles, cassoulets, vegetables, and all dishes that require long, slow simmering, either in the oven or on top of the stove. They are also referred to as saucepots, deep roasters with lids, and flameproof casseroles.

Dutch ovens can produce substantial whole-dish meals that soothe the spirits—homey, robust, comforting fare. These entrées can serve as the focal point of a meal, whether for a simple family supper or a casual company dinner.

It's only natural that many of these recipes encompass ethnic dishes as well as traditional classics that are kind to the budget and have been around for years. Favorites like Pork Ragout, Corned Beef with Onions and Greens, Irish Lamb Stew, Sweet-and-Sour Stuffed Cabbage, Osso Buco, Shrimp Jambalaya, Coq au Vin, Roasted Chicken with Garlic and Vegetables, Lamb Shanks Mediterranean, Belgian Beef Stew with Beer, Chicken Cacciatore, One-Pot Paella, Ham Hocks and Black-Eyed Peas—all can be found here.

The Dutch oven lends itself well to more wonderfully simple and rustic fare such as Lamb Meatball Stew with Barley, Chicken Breasts with Bulgur Wheat, Baked Apricot–Wild Rice Chicken, and Vegetable Chili.

So toss everything in the pot, put up your feet and relax, and let supper simmer.

1   MOM'S FAST CHILI
Prep: 10 minutes   Cook: 20 to 30 minutes   Serves: 6

This is a take-off on my mother's chili, which I grew up on. It's an old faithful in my weekly repertoire nowadays, and even better, it can be thrown together in a jiffy. You won't believe you can make chili so quickly. Serve topped with shredded cheddar cheese, shredded iceberg lettuce, chopped tomatoes, chopped onions, chopped avocado, and sour cream, if desired. To stretch chili for unexpected company, serve over rice.

1 pound lean ground beef	2½ teaspoons ground cumin
1 onion, chopped, or 2 tablespoons instant minced onion	1 (28-ounce) can crushed tomatoes with added puree
½ teaspoon garlic powder	1 (30-ounce) can chili beans
1 to 1½ tablespoons chili powder	1 (6-ounce) can tomato paste

1. In a large 4-quart Dutch oven or large saucepan, cook beef and onion over medium-high heat, stirring often to break up meat, until lightly browned, 5 to 10 minutes. Drain off excess fat.

2. Stir in all remaining ingredients. Heat to boiling. Reduce heat to medium-low and simmer, uncovered, 10 to 15 minutes.

2   CORNED BEEF WITH ONIONS AND GREENS
Prep: 20 minutes   Cook: 3 hours   Serves: 6 to 8

Instead of cabbage, try mustard or collard greens with your corned beef for an interesting change of pace.

1 (3-pound) corned beef	6 garlic cloves, mashed
2 tablespoons olive oil	¾ teaspoon pepper
4 large onions, sliced and separated into rings	2½ pounds potatoes, peeled and sliced ½ inch thick
1 (14½-ounce) can beef broth	1 bunch mustard or collard greens, shredded
1 (12-ounce) bottle dark beer	

1. Preheat oven to 325°. Rinse corned beef under cold water to remove spices; pat dry. In a 6-quart Dutch oven, heat oil over medium-high heat. Add corned beef, fat side down, and cook, turning once, until browned on both sides, 5 to 7 minutes. Remove to a cutting board and carve corned beef into ½-inch-thick slices.

2. In same pot, cook onions over medium heat, stirring occasionally, until golden, 3 to 5 minutes. Add broth, beer, garlic, and pepper. Layer corned beef slices and potato slices in onion-broth mixture.

3. Cover and bake 2½ hours. Add greens to pot. Cover and bake 15 minutes longer.

3 OVEN BEEF STEW
Prep: 10 minutes   Cook: 2½ hours   Serves: 6

Let this bake lazily in the oven while doing chores around the house.

3 pounds lean beef stew meat
   or boneless beef chuck
   roast, trimmed of fat and
   cut into 1-inch cubes
1 (10¾-ounce) can condensed
   cream of celery soup
½ (2.4-ounce) package dry leek
   soup mix

1 cup dry red wine
1 onion, coarsely chopped
5 medium baking potatoes,
   peeled and cut into
   eighths
8 carrots, peeled and halved
   crosswise
2 cups broccoli florets

1. Preheat oven to 350°. In 5-quart Dutch oven, combine beef, undiluted soup, dry soup mix, wine, and onion; mix well. Top with potato pieces and carrots, mixing in slightly. Cover and bake 2 hours.

2. Stir in broccoli, cover, and bake 15 minutes. Remove cover and bake 15 minutes longer.

4 BAKED BEEF AND EGGPLANT CASSEROLE
Prep: 15 minutes   Cook: 1¼ hours   Serves: 6

This shortcut eggplant casserole is easy to prepare.

1 pound lean ground beef
2 garlic cloves, minced
1 teaspoon salt
½ teaspoon pepper
½ cup long-grain white rice
2 pounds eggplant, cut into
   1-inch dice
2 tablespoons olive oil
2 teaspoons oregano

1 medium green bell pepper,
   sliced
1 medium onion, sliced
1 (28-ounce) can whole
   tomatoes, undrained and
   broken up
2 eggs, lightly beaten
1 tablespoon heavy cream

1. Preheat oven to 350°. In a 4-quart Dutch oven, cook beef with garlic, salt, and pepper, over medium-high heat, stirring often, until brown, 5 to 7 minutes. Drain off any fat.

2. Stir in rice and cook about 1½ minutes, or until translucent. Remove pan from heat.

3. Place eggplant over meat mixture. Drizzle 1 tablespoon oil over eggplant. Crush 1 teaspoon oregano between palms of hands and sprinkle over eggplant. Add a layer of green pepper and onion on top of eggplant. Add undrained tomatoes. Drizzle with remaining 1 tablespoon oil and sprinkle with remaining oregano.

4. Bake, covered, 1 hour, or until eggplant is completely cooked. Beat eggs with cream. Pour over casserole. Return to oven and bake 5 to 10 minutes, or until custard is set.

5 SPICY CABBAGE, BEEF, AND RICE
Prep: 20 minutes   Cook: 35 minutes   Serves: 6

An easy stove-top ground beef and rice dish zipped up with sausage and tomatoes with green chiles.

1 **pound lean ground beef**	1 **(10-ounce) can diced**
1 **pound smoked beef sausage**	**tomatoes and green chiles**
links, cut up	1 **teaspoon salt**
1 **cup long-grain white rice**	¼ **teaspoon cayenne**
1 **medium green bell pepper,**	1 **medium head green**
chopped	**cabbage, chopped**
1 **medium onion, chopped**	
1¾ **cups water**	

1. In a 5-quart Dutch oven, cook beef over medium-high heat, stirring occasionally, until meat loses its pink color, 5 to 7 minutes. Drain off any fat.

2. Add sausage and rice. Cook, stirring, until rice turns translucent, about 1½ minutes.

3. Stir in green pepper and onion and cook 1 minute. Stir in water, tomatoes with their liquid, salt, and cayenne. Heat to boiling.

4. Spread cabbage over meat mixture. Reduce heat to low, cover, and simmer 20 minutes. Stir cabbage down into dish and cook 5 minutes longer, or until rice is tender.

6 IRISH BEEF SHANKS
Prep: 20 minutes   Cook: 2½ hours   Serves: 4 to 6

This Irish rendition has plenty of hearty flavor with bacon and a bottle of good-quality dark beer.

6 **bacon slices**	¼ **teaspoon pepper**
6 **beef shanks, about 2½**	1 **onion, sliced**
pounds total	2 **carrots, peeled and sliced**
5 **tablespoons flour**	12 **small red potatoes (about 1**
1 **(12-ounce) bottle dark beer**	**pound)**
1 **(14½-ounce) can beef broth**	6 **garlic cloves, minced**
1 **(14½-ounce) can cut-up,**	½ **pound fresh mushrooms,**
peeled tomatoes,	**sliced**
undrained	10 **to 12 ounces sliced fresh**
1 **teaspoon allspice**	**spinach, cleaned and**
¼ **teaspoon salt**	**shredded**

1. Preheat oven to 325°. In a 5- or 6-quart Dutch oven, cook bacon over medium-high heat until very crisp, about 15 minutes. Remove with tongs and set aside.

2. In same pot, brown beef shanks in bacon drippings over medium-high heat, 7 to 8 minutes. Remove and set aside with bacon.

3. Add flour to drippings in pan and cook, stirring, over medium heat, for 1 minute. Add beer and broth and bring to a boil, whisking until thickened and smooth, 2 to 3 minutes. Add tomatoes with their liquid, allspice, salt, and pepper. Layer shanks, bacon, onion, carrots, potatoes, garlic, and mushrooms in gravy.

4. Cover and bake 2 hours. To serve, ladle shanks, vegetables, and gravy over shredded spinach in soup plates.

---

7 SWEET-AND-SOUR STUFFED CABBAGE
Prep: 20 minutes   Cook: 2¾ hours   Serves: 4

This old-fashioned recipe, shared by a friend, is reminiscent of one many of our mothers and grandmothers used to serve, including mine. With its old-world flavor, it's absolutely delicious and one of my favorites. Be sure to use ground beef sirloin to avoid excess fat in the finished dish.

1 large head green cabbage
1 pound ground beef sirloin
2 tablespoons finely minced onion
1 teaspoon salt
¼ teaspoon pepper
1 egg
1 tablespoon long-grain white rice

2 tablespoons water
1 (14½-ounce) can cut-up, peeled tomatoes, undrained
1 (15-ounce) can tomato sauce
½ cup packed brown sugar
⅓ cup fresh lemon juice
⅓ cup golden raisins

1. Preheat oven to 350°. Break off 8 larger outer leaves from head of cabbage. In a 4- or 5-quart Dutch oven half filled with boiling water, boil 8 leaves 4 to 6 minutes, just until they are pliable. Drain on paper towels; set aside.

2. Drain off all water and wipe out pot. In same pot, combine ground sirloin, onion, salt, pepper, egg, rice, and water; mix until well combined.

3. Arrange cabbage leaves on a flat surface with stem ends on the outside. Divide meat mixture evenly among the 8 leaves, placing near the stem end. Fold in sides over meat and carefully roll up.

4. Wash and dry the Dutch oven. Shred remaining cabbage and place in bottom of the same Dutch oven. Add tomatoes with their liquid, tomato sauce, brown sugar, lemon juice, and raisins; stir to blend well. Place cabbage rolls close together, seam side down, on top of tomato mixture. Spoon some of sauce on top and around cabbage rolls.

5. Cover and bake 2 hours. Remove lid and continue baking 30 minutes. To serve, place cabbage rolls on top of shredded cabbage.

8   SOUTHWESTERN BEEF STEW
Prep: 15 minutes   Cook: 2¾ hours   Serves: 6

Fix and forget this easy stove-top stew until the last half hour of cooking, when the lid of the cooking utensil should be removed to allow the juices to reduce to thicken the works.

2 tablespoons vegetable oil
2 pounds lean beef stew meat
   or round steak, cut into
   1-inch cubes
2 onions, chopped
2 large garlic cloves, crushed
   through a press
¾ pound fresh mushrooms,
   sliced
4 medium zucchini, sliced
1 red bell pepper, seeded and
   cut into thin strips

1 (16-ounce) package frozen
   corn kernels
1 cup chopped parsley
½ cup mild chile salsa
1 (28-ounce) can peeled whole
   tomatoes, drained and
   chopped
1 teaspoon oregano
¾ teaspoon ground cumin
¼ teaspoon crushed hot
   pepper flakes
¼ teaspoon salt

1. In a 5-quart Dutch oven or other large pot, heat oil until hot. Add beef and onions and cook over medium-high heat, stirring often, until beef is browned on all sides, 8 to 10 minutes.

2. Stir in all remaining ingredients; mix well. Heat to boiling, reduce heat, cover, and simmer 2 hours. Remove cover and simmer ½ hour longer, until meat is tender and pan juices are reduced slightly.

9   BELGIAN BEEF STEW WITH BEER
Prep: 15 minutes   Cook: 3 hours   Serves: 6

This hearty peasant-style stew is flavored throughout with onions and beer. To add color prior to serving, toss in some green vegetables and a cut-up fresh tomato. On a cold evening, serve with cooked noodles or plenty of crusty bread to sop up the good gravy.

1 (3-pound) boneless beef
   chuck roast
¼ teaspoon salt
¼ teaspoon pepper
¼ cup vegetable oil
4 onions, sliced
3 tablespoons flour
1 cup beef broth
1 (12-ounce) can beer

1 tablespoon white wine
   vinegar
½ teaspoon thyme
2 bay leaves
1 (9-ounce) package frozen cut
   Italian green beans
3 tablespoons chopped
   parsley

1. Cut beef into ½-inch-thick slices and season with salt and pepper. In a large flameproof casserole, heat 1 tablespoon oil. Add half of beef and cook over medium-high heat, turning, until browned, about 5 minutes. Remove to a plate. Repeat with another 1 tablespoon oil and remaining beef. Remove to a plate.

2. Add onions to any drippings remaining in pan. Cook, stirring often, until onions are tender and lightly browned, about 10 minutes. Remove to a plate. Add remaining 2 tablespoons oil to pan along with flour and cook, stirring, 1 minute.

3. Gradually whisk broth into flour mixture in pan, blending well. Stir in beer, vinegar, and thyme. Heat to boiling, stirring constantly. Reduce heat to low and add beef, onions, and bay leaves.

4. Cover and simmer 2 to 2½ hours, or until meat is tender. Last 10 minutes of cooking time, add green beans. To serve, remove bay leaves and garnish with parsley.

---

10   BAKED BEEF BRISKET WITH WHITE BEANS
Prep: 15 minutes   Cook: 3 to 3¼ hours   Serves: 6

Cook white beans alongside a fresh beef brisket in a tomato sauce mixture for a wonderful meal-in-a-dish. A splash of white wine and fresh basil add to the mélange of flavors and make the dish extra special.

2 **tablespoons vegetable oil**
2 **medium onions, chopped**
6 **medium carrots, peeled and chopped**
½ **cup chopped parsley**
3 **pounds fresh beef brisket (flat cut), trimmed of fat**
1 **(6-ounce) can tomato paste**
3 **cups water**
1 **teaspoon dry mustard**
2 **garlic cloves, minced**

1 **tablespoon brown sugar**
2 **tablespoons red wine vinegar**
1 **cup dried small white beans, rinsed and picked over**
1 **cup dry white wine**
1 **(9-ounce) package frozen Italian green beans**
⅓ **cup chopped fresh basil or parsley**

1. Preheat oven to 350°. In a 5- or 6-quart Dutch oven, heat oil over medium heat until hot. Add onions, carrots, and parsley. Cook, stirring often, until onions are golden, 8 to 10 minutes. Remove to a plate.

2. Add meat to pot and cook, turning, until brown on both sides, 6 to 8 minutes. Return carrots, onions and parsley to pot. Add tomato paste, water, mustard, garlic, brown sugar, vinegar, and white beans. Mix well. Heat to boiling.

3. Cover pot and transfer to oven. Bake 1½ hours.

4. Stir in wine. Cover and continue baking 1 to 1¼ hours, or until brisket and white beans are tender. Mix in green beans and basil. Return to oven and bake 15 minutes longer.

11   SUPER SPAGHETTI SAUCE
Prep: 10 minutes   Cook: 45 minutes   Serves: 12

This is the favorite spaghetti sauce in our house and its versatility is unbeatable. Serve immediately over hot cooked spaghetti or other pasta or hot steamed vegetables; or use sauce in making lasagne. Refrigerate any leftovers. This sauce also freezes well.

¾ **pound sweet or hot Italian sausage (or a combination of the two)**
1 **pound lean ground beef**
1 **large onion, chopped**
2 **garlic cloves, minced**
2 **(28-ounce) cans cut-up, peeled tomatoes, undrained**
¾ **cup dry white wine or dry vermouth**

1 **(12-ounce) can tomato paste**
1 **tablespoon Worcestershire sauce**
1 **teaspoon salt**
½ **teaspoon sugar**
2 **tablespoons chopped parsley**
2 **tablespoons dried basil**
½ **teaspoon fennel seeds**
¼ **teaspoon pepper**

1. Remove sausage from casings and crumble into a 5-quart Dutch oven. Add beef, onion, and garlic. Cook over medium-high heat, stirring often to break up lumps of meat, until browned, about 15 minutes. Drain off any fat.

2. Stir in tomatoes with their liquid, wine, tomato paste, Worcestershire sauce, salt, sugar, parsley, basil, fennel seeds, and pepper. Heat to boiling, stirring often. Reduce heat to low and simmer, uncovered, 30 minutes, stirring occasionally to prevent scorching.

12   SAUERBRATEN WITH CABBAGE AND SWEET POTATOES
Prep: 15 minutes   Cook: 1½ hours   Serves: 6 to 8

The sweet-and-sour flavors of sauerbraten are blended in this tasty stew chock-full of sweet potato and red cabbage pieces. Cider vinegar and gingersnap cookies in the gravy give it authentic flavor.

2 **tablespoons vegetable oil**
2 **pounds boneless beef chuck or beef top round steak, cut into 1-inch chunks**
2 **medium onions, coarsely chopped**
4 **medium to large sweet potatoes, peeled and cut into 2-inch chunks**
¾ **cup cider vinegar**

2 **cups water**
¼ **cup packed brown sugar**
2 **bay leaves**
5 **cups shredded red cabbage (about ½ medium head)**
5 **gingersnap cookies, crushed into fine crumbs (about ⅓ cup)**
⅓ **cup dark raisins**

1. In a 5-quart Dutch oven, heat 1 tablespoon oil over high heat until hot. Add half of beef and cook, stirring occasionally, until browned on all sides, about 5 minutes. With a slotted spoon, remove meat to a plate. Repeat procedure with remaining 1 tablespoon oil and remaining beef. Remove meat to same plate.

2. To drippings remaining in pot, add onions and cook until tender, about 5 minutes. Add sweet potatoes, vinegar, water, brown sugar, and bay leaves. Return beef to pot and mix in. Heat to boiling. Reduce heat to medium-low; cover and simmer 1 hour.

3. Stir in red cabbage, gingersnap crumbs, and raisins. Cover and simmer 20 to 25 minutes, or until cabbage is tender. Remove bay leaves before serving.

13   SPICED BEEF WITH WINTER VEGETABLES
Prep: 20 minutes   Cook: 3 hours   Serves: 6 to 8

This fabulous beef mélange, a favorite with all who taste it, is aromatic with cinnamon, nutmeg, ginger, and brandy and will warm the soul on a cold evening. Keep it in mind for casual holiday entertaining as well.

1 **(12-ounce) bottle dark beer**
1 **(14½-ounce) can beef broth**
½ **cup brandy**
1 **tablespoon Worcestershire sauce**
½ **cup quick-mixing flour**
1 **teaspoon ground cinnamon**
½ **teaspoon ground nutmeg**
½ **teaspoon ground ginger**
3 **tablespoons orange marmalade**
1 **teaspoon salt**
½ **teaspoon pepper**
2 **large onions, sliced and rings separated**
3 **large russet potatoes, peeled and sliced ½ inch thick**
3 **carrots, peeled and sliced ½ inch thick**
1 **cup pitted prunes**
½ **cup dried apricots**
2½ **pounds boneless beef chuck steaks, cut about 1 inch thick**

1. Preheat oven to 325°. In a deep 6-quart ovenproof casserole or Dutch oven, mix together beer, broth, brandy, Worcestershire sauce, flour, cinnamon, nutmeg, ginger, marmalade, salt, and pepper. Pour off 2 cups mixture into a measuring cup.

2. In broth mixture remaining in casserole, layer half of each of the following: onions, potatoes, carrots, prunes, and apricots. Place chuck steaks on top and repeat with a second layer, using remaining onions, potatoes, carrots, prunes, and apricots.

3. Pour reserved broth mixture over all. Cover and bake 2 hours. Uncover and ladle gravy from bottom of pan over top.

4. Cover, return to oven, and bake 1 hour longer.

14 ONE-POT PAELLA

Prep: 10 minutes   Cook: 1 hour   Serves: 6 to 8

This colorful dish would make appealing company fare.

1 tablespoon vegetable oil
8 chicken pieces (such as 2 thighs, 2 drumsticks, 4 breast halves)
½ pound turkey Italian sausage, sliced
2 medium onions, chopped
1 red bell pepper, cut into chunks
1 green bell pepper, cut into chunks
1½ cups converted rice
¾ teaspoon oregano

¼ teaspoon saffron threads, or ½ teaspoon ground turmeric
2 garlic cloves, crushed through a press
3 cups chicken broth
1 (16-ounce) package frozen peas, thawed
½ pound medium shrimp, shelled and deveined
½ cup canned quartered artichoke hearts, drained
2 tomatoes, cut into wedges

1. In a 5-quart Dutch oven, heat oil until hot. Add chicken pieces and cook over medium-high heat, turning, until brown on both sides, 5 to 7 minutes. Remove chicken to a plate. Add sausage to drippings and cook, stirring occasionally, until lightly browned, about 5 minutes; remove to a plate. Drain off all except 1 tablespoon pan drippings.

2. Add onions, red and green peppers, and rice. Cook over moderate heat, stirring constantly, 5 to 6 minutes, until onions are tender.

3. Stir in oregano, saffron, garlic, chicken broth, and cooked sausage. Heat to boiling.

4. Arrange chicken pieces on top of rice mixture. Reduce heat to low, cover, and simmer 30 minutes, or until most of liquid is absorbed and rice is tender.

5. Stir in peas, shrimp, and artichoke hearts. Cook until shrimp are pink, loosely curled, and opaque throughout, about 10 minutes longer. Gently stir in tomatoes. Serve hot.

15   BAKED APRICOT–WILD RICE CHICKEN
Prep: 15 minutes   Cook: 1¾ hours   Serves: 4 to 5

For best results, roast the chicken for an hour first and drain off all the fat and juices before adding the rice mixture.

1 (3-pound) broiler-fryer
    chicken
1 tablespoon honey
1 large onion, chopped
1 teaspoon minced garlic
½ teaspoon ground turmeric
    Juice of 1 lemon

1 (6.25-ounce) package quick-
    cooking long-grain and
    wild rice mix
1¾ cups hot water
½ cup dried apricots
½ cup pecan halves

1. Preheat oven to 350°. Clean chicken, discarding giblets and neck. Rinse cavity well and remove excess fat; pat dry. Tie legs together. Place chicken, breast side up, in a 5-quart Dutch oven.

2. Spread honey over chicken. Sprinkle with onion, garlic, turmeric, and lemon juice. Cover and bake 1 hour. Drain off all fat and liquid.

3. Sprinkle contents of rice and seasoning packets from rice mix around and under chicken. Pour water over rice. Add apricots. Cover and bake 35 to 45 minutes, or until rice is tender and chicken is cooked through.

4. Mix pecans into rice. Carve chicken into pieces and serve on top of rice.

16   CHICKEN BREASTS WITH BULGUR WHEAT
Prep: 15 minutes   Cook: 1½ hours   Serves: 6 to 8

This innovative dish couldn't be easier. Toss everything in a casserole, including frozen chicken tenders (do not thaw to avoid overcooking), pop into the oven, and relax until serving time.

1 (14½-ounce) can chicken
    broth
1 (28-ounce) can cut-up,
    peeled tomatoes,
    undrained
1 onion, coarsely chopped
3 garlic cloves, minced
    Juice and grated zest of
    1 lemon
½ cup slivered almonds

½ cup raisins
1 cup pimiento-stuffed green
    olives
½ teaspoon salt
¼ teaspoon pepper
2 cups bulgur
2 pounds frozen chicken
    breast tenders (do not
    thaw)

1. Preheat oven to 350°. In a 5-quart Dutch oven or casserole, combine all ingredients in order given. Stir to combine.

2. Cover and bake 1½ hours.

17 SIMPLE CASSOULET
Prep: 10 minutes   Cook: 2 hours   Serves: 6

A take-off of the classic French dish, this is a very simplified but wonderful tasting variation.

1 (1-pound) package dried
   Great Northern or navy
   beans, rinsed and picked
   over
5 cups water
1½ cups dry white wine
2 garlic cloves, minced
4 skinless, boneless chicken
   breast halves, quartered
½ pound Polish kielbasa
   sausage, cut into ¼-inch
   diagonal slices

¼ pound thinly sliced cooked
   ham, chopped
6 carrots, peeled and diced
4 celery ribs, chopped
1 large onion, chopped
1 teaspoon rosemary
1 teaspoon salt
½ teaspoon pepper
3 tablespoons chopped
   parsley

1. Preheat oven to 350°. In a 5-quart Dutch oven, combine beans and water; heat to boiling over high heat, stirring occasionally. Stir in wine, garlic, chicken, sausage, ham, carrots, celery, onion, rosemary, salt and pepper. Return to a boil.

2. Cover and bake 1½ hours. Remove cover and bake 15 to 20 minutes longer, or until beans are tender. Garnish with parsley.

18 CHICKEN CACCIATORE
Prep: 10 minutes   Cook: 1 hour   Serves: 4 to 5

Serve this wonderful classic saucy chicken dish over plenty of hot cooked pasta. Add Italian green beans the last few minutes of cooking time.

1 (3½- to 4-pound) broiler-
   fryer chicken, cut up
¼ teaspoon salt
¼ teaspoon pepper
¼ cup flour
2 tablespoons vegetable oil
2 onions, chopped
2 garlic cloves, minced
½ pound fresh mushrooms,
   sliced

1 (14½-ounce) can cut-up,
   peeled tomatoes,
   undrained
1 (8-ounce) can tomato sauce
2 teaspoons basil
¼ cup dry white wine
1 (9-ounce) package frozen cut
   Italian green beans

1. Season chicken pieces with salt and pepper. Sprinkle with 3 tablespoons flour to coat lightly.

2. In a 5-quart Dutch oven, heat oil. Add chicken and cook over medium-high heat, turning, until browned on both sides, 5 to 7 minutes. Remove to a plate.

3. In drippings remaining in pan, cook onions and garlic, stirring constantly, until onions are softened and light golden, about 5 minutes. Add mushrooms and cook, stirring, 3 minutes longer. Stir in remaining 1 tablespoon flour and cook, stirring, 1 minute longer, until thoroughly blended. Stir in tomatoes with their liquid, tomato sauce, and basil. Heat to boiling.

4. Return chicken to pan and spoon sauce over pieces. Cover and simmer over medium-low heat 35 minutes. Stir in wine and beans and simmer over low heat, uncovered, 10 minutes longer.

---

19 COQ AU VIN
Prep: 10 minutes   Cook: 50 to 56 minutes   Serves: 4 to 6

This classic dish can be made with your favorite chicken pieces. Add green beans so you have your vegetables and poultry cooked in a single pot.

8 bacon slices, diced	½ pound fresh mushrooms, stems trimmed
⅓ cup flour	8 carrots, peeled and diagonally sliced 1-inch thick
1 teaspoon salt	
½ teaspoon pepper	
½ teaspoon basil	
½ teaspoon thyme	2 cups dry red wine
½ teaspoon marjoram	1 tablespoon Dijon mustard
4 chicken breast halves, 2 chicken thighs, and 2 drumsticks, rinsed and drained	1 (9- or 10-ounce) package frozen green beans, thawed
16 to 20 small white onions, peeled	Chopped parsley, for garnish

1. In a 5-quart Dutch oven, cook bacon over medium heat until brown and crisp, about 5 minutes. With a slotted spoon, remove bacon bits to paper towels to drain.

2. Meanwhile, mix together flour, salt, pepper, basil, thyme, and marjoram. Dredge chicken all over in flour mixture. Shake off excess and reserve any remaining flour.

3. Cook chicken in 2 batches in hot bacon drippings over medium-high heat, turning, until golden, 5 to 7 minutes. Remove all chicken to a plate. Drain off any fat from pan.

4. Add onions, mushrooms, and carrots to brown bits in pan and cook, stirring, 2 minutes. Stir in any reserved flour and cook, stirring, 1 minute longer. Add wine, mustard, and bacon bits. Heat to boiling.

5. Return chicken to pan and bring to a boil. Reduce heat to low. Cover and simmer 30 to 35 minutes, or until chicken is done. Stir in green beans and cook 5 minutes longer. Garnish with a sprinkling of chopped parsley.

20   SAVORY CHICKEN SUNDAY SUPPER
Prep: 25 minutes   Cook: 30 to 40 minutes   Serves: 6

3 tablespoons vegetable oil
1 (2½- to 3-pound) broiler-
  fryer chicken, cut into
  pieces, skinned
1 medium onion, chopped
1 garlic clove, minced
½ cup finely chopped celery
  leaves
½ cup chopped green bell
  pepper

2 carrots, peeled and chopped
4 large red potatoes, peeled
  and cut into chunks
½ cup long-grain white rice
4 cups chicken broth
½ teaspoon marjoram
½ teaspoon salt
¼ teaspoon pepper
1 cup frozen peas, thawed

1. In a 5-quart Dutch oven, heat oil until hot over medium-high heat. Add chicken and cook, turning once, until golden on both sides, 8 to 10 minutes. Drain off any fat.

2. Add onion, garlic, celery leaves, green pepper, and carrots. Cook, stirring often, until onions are soft, 2 to 3 minutes.

3. Stir in potatoes, rice, broth, marjoram, salt, and pepper. Heat to boiling, reduce heat to low, and simmer, covered, until rice and potatoes are tender, 20 to 25 minutes. Stir in peas and let stand, covered, 5 minutes.

21   ROASTED CHICKEN WITH GARLIC AND VEGETABLES
Prep: 10 minutes   Cook: 1¾ hours   Serves: 4 to 6

This simple chicken dish is as wonderful looking as it is tasting. Don't be intimidated by the 40 garlic cloves. They don't overpower the dish. Once roasted, they become soft and make a great spread for French bread.

1 (4½- to 5-pound) roasting
  chicken
1 tablespoon vegetable oil
1 teaspoon paprika
40 garlic cloves, peeled
2 cups diagonally sliced
  peeled carrots (about 4)
4 baking potatoes, peeled and
  cut into eighths

2 celery ribs, cut diagonally
  into ½-inch slices
½ cup dry white wine
2 medium zucchini, sliced
3 pattypan squash, sliced
2 crookneck squash, sliced
  Fresh parsley, for garnish

1. Preheat oven to 375°. Rinse chicken inside and out; pat dry. Truss firmly with kitchen string.

2. Rub chicken with oil and sprinkle with paprika. Place breast side up in a 5-quart Dutch oven or roasting pan. Surround chicken with garlic cloves, carrots, potatoes, and celery. Pour wine over vegetables. Cover and bake 1 hour.

3. Remove cover. Place squash around sides of chicken. Return to oven and continue roasting, uncovered, 45 minutes longer, or until thigh juices run clear when pierced.

4. Arrange chicken on a heated serving platter and surround with garlic cloves and vegetables. Garnish with fresh parsley sprigs. If desired, skim fat from pan juices and pass separately. Spread garlic on French bread slices.

---

22   SAN PASQUAL STEW
Prep: 20 minutes   Cook: 2 hours   Serves: 6 to 8

Named after the street on which the super cook who developed this dish lives in Southern California, this recipe is guaranteed to be a surefire hit.

1 (1-pound) package dried
   pinto beans, rinsed and
   picked over
3 pounds beef short ribs
2 onions, coarsely chopped
1½ tablespoons garlic powder
2 quarts water
4 skinless, boneless chicken
   breast halves, each cut
   into 4 or 5 pieces
1 (28-ounce) can cut-up,
   peeled tomatoes,
   undrained
1 (4-ounce) can diced green
   chiles

1 (15-ounce) can golden
   hominy, drained
½ head Napa cabbage, finely
   shredded (about 4 cups)
½ teaspoon salt
½ teaspoon pepper
¼ to ½ teaspoon cayenne
   Shredded Monterey Jack
   cheese, chopped cilantro,
   chopped scallions, salsa,
   and bread or tortillas, as
   accompaniment

1. Place beans in a 6-quart Dutch oven. Add ribs, onions, garlic powder, and water. Heat to boiling over high heat. Reduce heat to medium-low, cover, and simmer 1½ hours.

2. Stir in chicken, tomatoes with their juices, and chiles. Cover and cook 15 minutes.

3. With the back of a large spoon or a potato masher, mash some of pinto beans in pot to thicken stew. Stir in hominy, cabbage, salt, pepper, and cayenne. Turn off heat, cover, and let stand 5 minutes. Serve with cheese, cilantro, scallions, salsa, and bread or tortillas.

23   NOODLE-RICE CHICKEN BAKE
Prep: 15 minutes   Cook: 50 minutes   Serves: 10

Another tried-and-true recipe shared by a friend, this one is great for a crowd. It's an excellent way to use leftover cooked poultry.

1   stick (¼ pound) butter
1   (12-ounce) package very fine
      egg noodles
2   cups quick-cooking long-
      grain white rice
1   cup water
1   tablespoon soy sauce
2   (14½-ounce) cans chicken
      broth

2   (10½-ounce) cans French
      onion soup
1   (8-ounce) can sliced water
      chestnuts, drained
3   cups diced cooked chicken
1   (16-ounce) package frozen
      peas

1. Preheat oven to 350°. In a 5-quart Dutch oven, melt butter over medium heat. Add noodles and cook, stirring constantly, until noodles are crisp and light brown, about 5 minutes.

2. Add rice, water, soy sauce, broth, undiluted onion soup, water chestnuts, and chicken. Mix well.

3. Cover and bake 40 minutes. Mix in peas, cover, and bake 5 to 7 minutes longer, or until peas are hot and tender.

24   ORANGE CHICKEN WITH BROCCOLI
Prep: 10 minutes   Cook: 50 to 55 minutes   Serves: 5 to 6

Chicken with citrus and broccoli is a refreshing change-of-pace offering.

1   (3- to 3½-pound) chicken,
      cut up
2   tablespoons flour
½   teaspoon salt
¼   teaspoon ground cinnamon
2   tablespoons vegetable oil
1   medium onion, chopped
1   cup converted rice

2   cups orange juice
¼   teaspoon hot pepper sauce
6   carrots, peeled and cut into
      1-inch slices
1   bunch broccoli, cut into
      florets (4 cups)
1   navel orange, sliced

1. Remove fat from chicken; remove skin, if desired. Rinse chicken and pat dry with paper towels. Mix together flour, salt, and cinnamon. Dredge chicken pieces in seasoned flour.

2. In a 5-quart Dutch oven, heat oil over medium-high heat until hot. Add chicken pieces, and cook, turning, until well browned all over, 5 to 7 minutes. Cover and cook chicken over medium-high heat about 10 minutes, turning once, to cook part way through. Remove chicken to a plate. Drain fat from pan.

3. Add onion and rice to pan and cook, stirring, 3 minutes. Stir in orange juice, hot sauce, and carrots. Heat to boiling over high heat. Return chicken to pan, placing on top of rice mixture. Reduce heat to medium-low, cover, and simmer 20 minutes.

4. Add broccoli and orange slices. Cover and cook 10 to 15 minutes longer, until rice and broccoli are tender.

---

25 PHILIPPINE-STYLE STEW
Prep: 15 minutes   Cook: 1 hour   Serves: 6 to 8

A Philippine knife-and-fork stew known as *pochero* was the inspiration for this dish.

10 ounces chorizo sausages, casings removed
1 medium onion, chopped
5 garlic cloves, mashed
1 (14½-ounce) can chicken broth
1 (14½-ounce) can cut-up, peeled tomatoes, undrained
3 cups water
1 bay leaf
½ teaspoon ground ginger
2 whole skinless, boneless chicken breasts, or 4 halves (about 1½ pounds), cut into 1½-inch chunks

1 (8¾-ounce) can garbanzo beans (chick-peas), drained
2 sweet potatoes, peeled and sliced ½ inch thick
1 cup converted rice
½ pound bok choy, washed and shredded (both tops and stalks)
2 firm bananas, sliced
3 scallions, sliced

1. In a 6-quart Dutch oven, break up chorizo with a spoon and cook over medium heat, stirring occasionally, 5 minutes. Add onion and cook, stirring, until softened, 2 to 3 minutes.

2. Stir in garlic, chicken broth, tomatoes with their liquid, water, bay leaf, ginger, chicken, garbanzo beans, sweet potatoes, and rice. Heat to simmering over medium-high heat. Reduce heat to medium-low. Cover and simmer 40 minutes.

3. Stir in bok choy and bananas. Cover and cook 10 to 15 minutes. Serve in bowls, with a sprinkling of scallions.

26   CHICKEN POTATO STEW
Prep: 20 minutes   Cook: 40 to 45 minutes   Serves: 6

This hearty variation of a festive South American dish is usually served during the Christmas holidays.

1 (2½- to 3-pound) chicken, cut up
2 tablespoons vegetable oil
2 scallions, chopped
¼ cup chopped cilantro
2 tablespoons chopped parsley
2 cups chicken broth
1 teaspoon ground cumin
1 teaspoon salt
¼ teaspoon pepper
½ pound carrots, peeled and diced
2 pounds russet potatoes, peeled and cut into 1-inch cubes
2 cups corn kernels
3 tablespoons drained capers
½ cup heavy cream

1. Rinse and dry chicken. In a 5-quart Dutch oven, heat oil over high heat until hot. Add chicken pieces and cook, turning until golden, 6 to 8 minutes. Drain off any fat.

2. Add scallions, 2 tablespoons cilantro, and the parsley. Cook, stirring 1 minute.

3. Mix in chicken broth, cumin, salt, and pepper. Heat to boiling, reduce heat to low, cover, and simmer 10 minutes. Stir in carrots and potatoes. Simmer, covered, 10 minutes.

4. Stir in corn, capers, and cream. Simmer, uncovered, until potatoes and carrots are tender and sauce has thickened slightly, 10 to 15 minutes. Garnish with remaining 2 tablespoons cilantro.

27   TURKEY BLACK BEAN CHILI
Prep: 5 minutes   Cook: 35 minutes   Serves: 6 to 8

Try this interesting combination for a change. It goes together effortlessly with canned black beans. Of course, if you feel so inclined you can cook dried black beans to use in this dish.

1 pound ground turkey
1 onion, chopped
1 tablespoon vegetable oil
2 large garlic cloves, crushed through a press
1½ tablespoons chili powder
½ teaspoon salt
1 (4-ounce) can diced green chiles
2 (28-ounce cans) crushed tomatoes with added puree
2 (16-ounce) cans black beans, rinsed and drained
Optional accompaniments: Sour cream, shredded cheddar cheese, chopped scallions, and guacamole

1. In a large pot, cook turkey and onion in oil over medium-high heat, stirring to break up lumps, until turkey is no longer pink, 5 to 7 minutes. Drain off any excess fat.

2. Add all remaining ingredients; stir to mix well. Heat to boiling, stirring often. Reduce heat to low and simmer, stirring occasionally, 30 minutes. Serve topped with sour cream, shredded cheddar cheese, chopped scallions, and guacamole, if desired.

28 PICADILLO
Prep: 10 minutes   Cook: 20 to 25 minutes   Serves: 6

This is a great buffet offering for an informal party, with hot cooked rice on the side. It can also be frozen for 2 to 3 months. Our tasters loved the somewhat exotic flavor. The recipe can be doubled or tripled for a larger crowd.

1½ pounds ground turkey or
    lean ground beef
1 tablespoon olive oil
2 garlic cloves, crushed
    through a press
1 large onion, chopped
1 green bell pepper, chopped
1 (14½-ounce) can cut-up,
    peeled tomatoes,
    undrained
1 (6-ounce) can tomato paste
½ cup dry sherry
½ teaspoon ground cumin

½ teaspoon chili powder
¼ teaspoon dry mustard
⅛ teaspoon ground cinnamon
    Pinch of ground cloves
¾ teaspoon salt
¼ teaspoon pepper
1 tablespoon brown sugar
½ cup raisins
½ cup coarsely chopped
    pimiento-stuffed green
    olives
½ cup slivered almonds,
    toasted

1. In a 4- or 5-quart flameproof casserole, cook meat in oil over medium-high heat, stirring to break up lumps, until browned, 5 to 7 minutes. (If using beef, drain off excess fat.)

2. Add garlic, onion, and green pepper. Cook, stirring often, until onion is tender, about 3 minutes.

3. Stir in all remaining ingredients except almonds. Heat to boiling, stirring occasionally. Reduce heat to low and simmer, uncovered, 15 to 20 minutes. Serve hot, garnished with almonds.

29   TURKEY AND SQUASH STEW

Prep: 10 minutes   Cook: 1¼ hours   Serves: 5 to 6

Squash combines with cinnamon, brown sugar, and wine to make this interesting stove-top dish using a turkey breast.

6 bacon slices, chopped	2 tablespoons chopped
3 tablespoons flour	parsley
1 (2- to 2½-pound) turkey	1 cup white wine
breast half, skin removed	⅓ cup water
1 medium onion, coarsely	5 cups 1½-inch cubes skinned
chopped	Hubbard squash (about 2
4 celery ribs, chopped	pounds)
4 carrots, peeled and chopped	½ teaspoon ground cinnamon
	2 tablespoons brown sugar

1. In a 5- or 6-quart Dutch oven, fry bacon over medium-high heat until crisp. Remove bacon to a plate. Drain off all except 2 tablespoons drippings from pot.

2. Sprinkle flour over turkey to coat. Cook, turning, until golden on both sides. Remove turkey to a plate.

3. Add onion, celery, and carrots to pot. Cook until onion is limp, about 3 minutes. Stir in parsley, wine, and water. Mix well. Return turkey to pot. Add squash. Heat to boiling. Reduce heat to medium, cover, and simmer 1 hour to 1 hour and 10 minutes, or until turkey is cooked through.

4. Stir in cinnamon and brown sugar. Heat to boiling, stirring occasionally. Reduce heat and simmer 3 minutes. Stir in bacon. Slice turkey and serve with vegetables and sauce mixture.

30   HAM HOCKS AND BLACK-EYED PEAS

Prep: 10 minutes   Cook: 2 to 2½ hours   Serves: 4 to 5

This is inexpensive hearty fare that warms the soul. A bowl of this is a cross between a soup and stew.

1 pound dried black-eyed	1 celery rib, chopped
peas	3 cups water
1 green bell pepper, chopped	2 cups packed chopped
1 red bell pepper, chopped	collard greens
1 onion, chopped	3 pounds smoked ham hocks

1. In a large flameproof casserole, combine all ingredients except ham hocks and heat to boiling, stirring occasionally.

2. Place ham hocks on top of mixture and reduce heat to low. Cover and simmer 2 to 2½ hours, or until beans and ham hocks are tender.

31 CURRIED HAM AND RICE
Prep: 15 minutes   Cook: 35 minutes   Serves: 8 to 10

This is a family favorite my mother has been making for years. It's great without the meat as an accompaniment for baked ham as well. Either way, the leftovers are wonderful reheated in a microwave oven.

1 stick (¼ pound) butter
1 large onion, sliced
2 cups converted rice
4 cups boiling water
1 teaspoon curry powder
½ teaspoon ground cumin
⅛ teaspoon cayenne
⅛ teaspoon turmeric
⅛ teaspoon ground ginger
½ teaspoon salt

⅛ teaspoon pepper
1 (16-ounce) package frozen peas, thawed
3 cups diced cooked ham
Chopped scallions, mango chutney, chopped roasted peanuts, raisins, and shredded coconut, as accompaniment

1. In a 4- or 5-quart Dutch oven, melt butter over medium-high heat. Add onion and cook, stirring, until softened, 3 to 4 minutes. Add rice and cook, stirring, until rice turns translucent, about 5 minutes.

2. Stir in boiling water, curry powder, cumin, cayenne, turmeric, ginger, salt, and pepper. Heat to boiling and reduce heat to low. Cover tightly and simmer 25 minutes, or until all liquid is absorbed.

3. Stir in peas and ham. Cover and cook over medium-low heat 5 to 7 minutes, or until peas and ham are hot. Pass condiments such as chopped scallions, chutney, chopped peanuts, raisins, and shredded coconut, if desired.

CURRIED SHRIMP AND RICE

Substitute 1¼ pounds cooked, shelled, and deveined medium shrimp for ham and stir in ½ cup chopped roasted red pepper along with shrimp.

CURRIED CHICKEN AND RICE

Substitute 3 cups diced cooked chicken for ham and stir in ½ cup chopped red bell pepper along with chicken.

32   BARBECUED LIMAS AND HAM
Prep: 15 minutes   Cook: 3¼ hours   Serves: 6

A wonderful old-fashioned barbecued bean dish that rates raves.

½   pound salt pork
1   (1-pound) package large
      dried lima beans, rinsed
      and picked over
1   large onion, chopped
5   garlic cloves, mashed
4   cups water
½   pound cooked ham, cut into
      ¾-inch cubes
1   medium green bell pepper,
      chopped
1   (14½-ounce) can cut-up,
      peeled tomatoes,
      undrained

1   tablespoon chili powder
1   tablespoon prepared yellow
      mustard
1   tablespoon Worcestershire
      sauce
1   teaspoon paprika
½   teaspoon ground allspice
¼   cup molasses
¼   cup packed brown sugar
¼   cup red wine vinegar
1   (6-ounce) can tomato paste
½   teaspoon pepper

1. Rinse salt pork to remove excess salt. Partially cut crosswise at ½-inch intervals, being careful not to cut through rind.

2. In a 5-quart flameproof casserole, cook salt pork, fat side down, over high heat until browned on bottom, 3 to 5 minutes.

3. Remove pan from heat. Stir in beans, onion, garlic, and water. Heat to boiling, reduce heat to medium-low, cover, and cook 1½ hours.

4. Preheat oven to 350°. Add ham, green pepper, tomatoes with their liquid, chili powder, mustard, Worcestershire sauce, paprika, allspice, molasses, brown sugar, vinegar, tomato paste, and pepper to bean mixture; mix thoroughly. Cover. Transfer to oven and bake 1½ hours, or until beans are tender.

33   LAMB RIBLETS, SOUTHWESTERN STYLE
Prep: 15 minutes   Cook: 35 to 40 minutes   Serves: 6 to 7

2   tablespoons olive oil
2½ pounds lamb riblets
1   medium green bell pepper,
      chopped
1   medium red bell pepper,
      chopped
1   medium red onion, chopped
2   cups converted rice

2   (14½-ounce) cans chicken
      broth
1   (4-ounce) can diced green
      chiles
1   teaspoon ground cumin
1   teaspoon oregano
½   teaspoon salt
¼   teaspoon pepper

1. In a 4½-quart Dutch oven or deep 12-inch skillet, heat oil over medium-high heat until hot. Add riblets and cook, turning, until browned on both sides, 5 to 7 minutes. Remove and set aside.

2. In same pan, cook green and red peppers and red onion over medium heat, stirring occasionally, 2 to 3 minutes, or until soft. Stir in rice, broth, chiles, cumin, oregano, salt, and pepper. Heat to boiling, reduce heat to low, then top with riblets. Cover and simmer 25 minutes.

34   LAMB SHANKS MEDITERRANEAN
Prep: 25 minutes   Cook: 3½ hours   Serves: 4

Once considered a humble cut of meat, lamb shanks are no longer inexpensive. You can simmer the shanks a day in advance, refrigerate, and reheat on top of the stove just before serving. This dish is appealingly rustic, good company fare.

2 tablespoons olive oil	1 teaspoon mint
4 (1-pound) lamb shanks	1 (8-ounce) can tomato sauce
2 medium onions, chopped	1 cup dry white wine
2 medium zucchini, chopped	3 tablespoons fresh lemon
6 medium carrots, pared and	juice
chopped	1 (6-ounce) can pitted whole
2 garlic cloves, crushed	ripe olives, drained
2 teaspoons basil	½ teaspoon pepper
1 teaspoon oregano	

1. In a large flameproof casserole, heat 1 tablespoon oil over medium-high heat until hot. Add 2 lamb shanks and cook, turning, until well browned all over. Remove shanks to a plate. Repeat with remaining 1 tablespoon oil and remaining lamb shanks; remove shanks to a plate.

2. Drain off all but 1 tablespoon drippings in pan. Add onions and cook over medium heat, stirring often, until golden, about 8 minutes. Stir in zucchini and carrots and cook, stirring, 2 to 3 minutes. Stir in garlic, basil, oregano, mint, tomato sauce, and wine. Heat to boiling. Add lamb shanks, pushing them into sauce mixture. Cover, reduce heat to medium-low, and simmer 3 to 3½ hours, until lamb is very tender and falls away from bone.

3. Stir in lemon juice, olives, and pepper. Serve over or alongside hot cooked corkscrew pasta or orzo. Garnish with lemon slices, if desired.

35 LAMB CHOPS WITH RATATOUILLE AND COUSCOUS

Prep: 15 minutes   Cook: 45 to 50 minutes   Serves: 6

This recipe is drenched with Mediterranean flavor and flair.

3 tablespoons olive oil
6 shoulder lamb chops or leg
   steaks (about 2½ pounds)
1 large onion, halved and cut
   into ½-inch-thick slices
1 large red bell pepper, cut
   into ¼-inch strips
3 medium zucchini, cut into
   ½-inch-thick slices
5 large garlic cloves, mashed
1 (1-pound) eggplant, peeled
   and cut into ½-inch cubes

1 (28-ounce) can cut-up,
   peeled tomatoes,
   undrained
1 cup dry white wine
1 teaspoon oregano
1 teaspoon basil
1 (10-ounce) package couscous
½ cup small pimiento-stuffed
   green olives
1 teaspoon salt
½ teaspoon pepper

1. In a 4-quart flameproof casserole, heat oil over high heat. Add chops and brown on both sides, 2 or 3 at a time, a total of about 5 minutes. Remove to a dish and set aside.

2. Reduce heat to medium-high, and in same casserole, cook onion and red pepper, stirring often, 2 minutes. Add zucchini, garlic, eggplant, tomatoes with their liquid, wine, oregano, basil, couscous, green olives, salt, and pepper. Mix well. Heat to boiling. Place lamb on top of vegetable mixture, reduce heat to low, cover, and cook 30 to 35 minutes, or until lamb is cooked to desired doneness.

36 IRISH LAMB STEW

Prep: 25 minutes   Cook: 2 hours 20 minutes   Serves: 6 to 8

This is an appealing, soul-warming rendition of a classic dish.

6 bacon slices
5 tablespoons olive oil
2 pounds boneless leg of
   lamb, cubed
½ cup flour
1 (14½-ounce) can beef broth
1 (28-ounce) can cut-up,
   peeled tomatoes,
   undrained
½ teaspoon paprika
½ teaspoon ground mace

1 tablespoon Worcestershire
   sauce
1 teaspoon salt
½ teaspoon pepper
3 garlic cloves, minced
1 large onion, sliced
2 carrots, peeled and sliced
3 large potatoes, peeled and
   cubed (about 2½ pounds)
1 (10-ounce) package frozen
   peas

1. Preheat oven to 350°. In a 5- or 6-quart Dutch oven, cook bacon over medium heat until crisp, about 10 minutes. Remove bacon; drain off and discard fat.

2. Heat olive oil in same pot over high heat. Add lamb and cook, turning, until browned on all sides, 5 to 7 minutes. Remove lamb.

3. Reduce heat to medium-high, add flour to pan, and cook, stirring, 1 minute. Add broth and bring to a boil, whisking until thickened and smooth, 1 to 2 minutes.

4. Stir in tomatoes with their juice, paprika, mace, Worcestershire sauce, salt, pepper, garlic, onion, carrots, and potatoes. Mix well. Return lamb and bacon to pot. Cover and bake 1 hour and 55 minutes.

5. Add peas. Cover and let stand 5 minutes.

---

37 LAMB MEATBALL STEW WITH BARLEY
Prep: 30 minutes   Cook: 1¾ hours   Serves: 6 to 8

This is truly wonderful tasting comfort food.

1½ **pounds ground lamb**	1 **large carrot, peeled and**
1 **teaspoon dried mint**	**diced**
½ **cup Italian seasoned bread**	1 **small turnip, peeled and**
crumbs	**diced**
1 **egg**	2 **celery ribs, diced**
½ **teaspoon garlic salt**	3 **garlic cloves, minced**
¼ **teaspoon pepper**	1 **cup pearl barley**
2 **(14½-ounce) cans chicken**	¼ **cup chopped parsley**
broth	**Juice and grated zest of**
1 **(8¾-ounce) can kidney**	**1 lemon**
beans, rinsed and drained	**Salt**
1 **(28-ounce) can cut-up,**	
peeled tomatoes,	
undrained	

1. In a 5- to 6-quart Dutch oven, combine lamb, mint, bread crumbs, egg, garlic salt, and pepper. Using your hands, mix ingredients together well. Form into 1½-inch meatballs and set aside on wax paper.

2. In same pan, combine chicken broth, kidney beans, tomatoes with their liquid, carrot, turnip, celery, garlic, and barley. Stir to mix. Heat to boiling; reduce heat to low. Carefully add meatballs. Cover and simmer 1½ hours. Stir in parsley, lemon juice, and lemon zest. Taste and season with salt and additional pepper, if necessary.

38   ONE-POT MEATLESS CHILI
Prep: 5 minutes   Cook: 20 minutes   Serves: 4

When you're in a hurry and want to get something on the table fast, try this dish made mostly with items more than likely on your pantry shelf.

1   tablespoon vegetable oil
1   medium onion, chopped
3   garlic cloves, minced
¼   cup canned diced green chiles
2   to 2½ tablespoons chili powder
1   (28-ounce) can cut-up peeled tomatoes, undrained
1   (15-ounce) can pinto beans, rinsed and drained
1   (15-ounce) can Great Northern beans, rinsed and drained
1   cup frozen or canned corn kernels
½   teaspoon salt
¼   teaspoon pepper
    Grated cheddar or Monterey Jack cheese, plain yogurt, and chopped fresh cilantro or scallion green, for garnish

1. In large flameproof casserole or nonreactive saucepan, heat oil until hot. Add onion and garlic and cook over medium heat, stirring, until onion is soft, about 5 minutes.

2. Stir in chiles, chili powder, tomatoes with their liquid, beans, corn, salt, and pepper. Heat to boiling, stirring. Reduce heat to low and simmer, uncovered, 10 minutes.

3. Serve topped with cheese, yogurt, and cilantro.

39   BURRITOS RANCHEROS
Prep: 20 minutes   Cook: 3 to 3½ hours   Serves: 6 to 8

1   (3- to 4-pound) beef chuck roast
2   tablespoons chili powder
1   teaspoon oregano
¼   teaspoon ground cumin
2   garlic cloves, crushed through a press
1   Anaheim, or other semi-hot green chile, seeded and chopped
2   medium onions, chopped
1   (28-ounce) can cut-up, peeled tomatoes, undrained
1   (30-ounce) can chili beans, drained
2½   to 3 tablespoons quick-mixing flour
3   tablespoons cold water
8   flour tortillas, warmed
1   cup shredded cheddar cheese (4 ounces)
    Guacamole Supreme (recipe follows)
¾   cup sour cream

1. In a 6-quart Dutch oven, brown beef on both sides over high heat. Add chili powder, oregano, cumin, garlic, chile, and onions.

2. Stir in tomatoes with their liquid. Heat to boiling; reduce heat to low and cook 2½ to 3 hours, or until meat falls apart. Remove meat from cooking liquid and let stand until cool enough to handle easily.

3. Add beans. Blend together flour and cold water and stir into liquid in pot. Heat to boiling, stirring. Reduce heat to low and simmer 5 minutes.

4. Shred meat with a fork, discarding any fat and bones. Return meat to pot and simmer 5 minutes.

5. Spoon some of meat and bean mixture down center of each tortilla. Fold in ends and roll up. Place seam side down on a plate and top with more hot meat mixture. Top with cheese, Guacamole Supreme, and sour cream.

GUACAMOLE SUPREME

Mash 2 large ripe avocados with a fork. Blend in ½ teaspoon seasoned salt, 1 garlic clove, minced, 1 teaspoon minced fresh cilantro (optional), and 2 tablespoons fresh lime juice.

40 VEGETABLE CHILI
Prep: 30 minutes   Cook: 45 to 50 minutes   Serves: 5 to 6

You'll never miss the meat in this wonderful mélange of vegetables with chililike taste and texture. The dish can stand alone or you can top it with shredded cheese, if desired.

2 tablespoons vegetable oil
1 medium onion, chopped
4 yellow crookneck squash, cut into ½-inch dice (3 cups)
1 large zucchini, cut into ½-inch dice
1 medium red bell pepper, coarsely chopped
1 medium green bell pepper, coarsely chopped
2 celery ribs, chopped
1 cup quartered fresh mushrooms
3 carrots, peeled and chopped
2 large tomatoes, chopped
1 (16-ounce) package frozen black-eyed peas
½ cup dry white wine
1 (6-ounce) can tomato paste
1½ tablespoons chili powder
1½ teaspoons ground cumin
1 teaspoon minced garlic
1 teaspoon salt
¼ teaspoon pepper
1 cup shredded cheddar cheese (optional)

1. In a 5-quart pot, heat oil over medium-high heat. Add onion and cook, stirring often, until softened, 2 to 3 minutes.

2. Add yellow squash, zucchini, red and green pepper, celery, mushrooms, and carrots. Cook, stirring often, until vegetables are crisp-tender, 8 to 10 minutes.

3. Stir in tomatoes, peas, wine, tomato paste, chili powder, cumin, garlic, salt, and pepper. Mix well. Heat to boiling, reduce heat to medium-low, cover, and simmer 20 to 25 minutes, stirring occasionally, until vegetables are tender. Top with shredded cheddar cheese, if desired.

41   RATATOUILLE SUPREME
Prep: 10 minutes   Cook: 35 minutes   Serves: 5 to 6

This is a great vegetarian main dish, served hot or chilled. If desired, top while hot with shredded cheese. Another time, add cubed cooked meat and serve hot over rice, in pita bread, or rolled up in flour tortillas, burrito style.

3 tablespoons olive oil
2 onions, chopped
2 large garlic cloves, crushed
   through a press
1 medium eggplant (1 to 1¼
   pounds), cut into 1-inch
   dice
1 medium green bell pepper,
   cut into 1-inch squares
1 medium red bell pepper, cut
   into 1-inch squares
6 medium zucchini, sliced

3 medium tomatoes,
   chopped, or 1 (14-ounce)
   can whole peeled
   tomatoes, drained and
   chopped
½ cup chopped parsley
¼ cup chopped fresh basil
½ teaspoon seasoned salt
¼ teaspoon pepper
2 tablespoons tomato paste
1 cup shredded cheddar,
   Gruyère, or Fontina
   cheese

1. In 4- or 5-quart Dutch oven or large pot, heat oil until hot. Add onions, garlic, eggplant, and peppers and cook over medium heat, stirring often, until onions are crisp-tender, about 5 minutes.

2. Stir in zucchini, tomatoes, parsley, and basil. Heat to boiling. Reduce heat to medium, cover, and cook 15 minutes.

3. Remove cover and stir in seasoned salt and pepper. Continue cooking, uncovered, 10 minutes longer. Stir in tomato paste. Serve as is or over hot cooked rice. Top each serving with a sprinkling of shredded cheese.

TURKEY OR CHICKEN RATATOUILLE

Stir in 2 to 3 cups chopped cooked turkey or chicken with the seasoned salt and pepper. Proceed as recipe directs. Serve in pita bread, over hot cooked rice, or rolled up in a flour tortilla.

42   BOUILLABAISSE
Prep: 10 minutes   Cook: 1¾ hours   Serves: 6 to 8

This is a versatile dish for your entertaining repertoire. Make the base in advance and freeze, if desired. Heat it and toss in your favorite kinds of fish 15 minutes prior to serving. Be sure to pass plenty of crusty French bread.

¼ cup olive oil
1 large leek (white and tender green), washed well and chopped
1 large onion, chopped
1 large carrot, peeled and chopped
5 garlic cloves, minced
2 celery ribs, sliced
1 small fennel bulb (about ½ pound), finely chopped, green fronds reserved
1 (28-ounce) can cut-up, peeled tomatoes, undrained

2 (14 ½-ounce) cans chicken broth
½ pound peeled and deveined shrimp
1 pound skinless, boneless firm white fish (such as halibut, cod, or swordfish), cut into 1-inch cubes
½ pound scallops
1 pound clams, scrubbed
Salt and pepper
Rouille (recipe follows)

1. In a 5- or 6-quart Dutch oven, heat oil until hot over medium-high heat. Add leek, onion, carrot, garlic, celery, and fennel bulb. Cook, stirring occasionally, until lightly browned, 5 to 7 minutes.

2. Stir in tomatoes with their liquid and broth. Cover and cook over medium-low heat 1½ hours. (The stock can be refrigerated or frozen at this point.)

3. Add shrimp, fish, scallops, and clams and cook, covered, over medium heat 5 to 10 minutes, until shrimp are pink, scallops and fish are white throughout, and clams open. (Discard any clams that do not open.) Season with salt and pepper to taste. Serve in soup bowls, topped with sprigs of green fennel fronds. Pass Rouille to spoon on top.

ROUILLE

In a food processor fitted with the metal blade, combine 3 tablespoons olive oil, ¼ cup bread crumbs, 3 garlic cloves, minced, 2 tablespoons basil, 1 (2-ounce) jar sliced pimientos, ¼ teaspoon salt, and ⅛ teaspoon cayenne. Process until mixture is smooth.

43   SHRIMP JAMBALAYA
Prep: 15 minutes   Cook: 45 minutes   Serves: 6

2 tablespoons butter or
   margarine
2 medium onions, chopped
2 green bell peppers, chopped
3 celery ribs, chopped
3 ounces cooked ham,
   chopped (about 1 cup)
2 garlic cloves, crushed
   through a press
1½ cups converted rice
1½ cups beef broth

1 (28-ounce) can cut-up,
   peeled tomatoes,
   undrained
3 tablespoons chopped
   parsley
1 teaspoon basil
½ teaspoon thyme
¼ teaspoon pepper
⅛ teaspoon cayenne
1 pound medium shrimp,
   shelled and deveined

1. In a 5-quart Dutch oven or pot, melt butter over medium heat. Add onions, green peppers, celery, ham, and garlic. Cook, stirring occasionally, until vegetables are soft, about 5 minutes.

2. Add rice and cook, stirring often, 3 minutes. Stir in broth, tomatoes with their liquid, 2 tablespoons parsley, basil, thyme, pepper, and cayenne. Heat to boiling. Reduce heat to low, cover, and simmer 25 minutes.

3. Stir in shrimp and cook about 10 minutes longer, or until shrimp are opaque throughout and rice is tender and liquid is absorbed. Garnish with remaining 1 tablespoon chopped parsley.

44   MUSSELS MARINARA
Prep: 20 minutes   Cook: 20 minutes   Serves: 3 to 4

Here's a wonderful Italian-inspired way to serve fresh mussels. Be sure to have plenty of crusty bread handy for dipping in the sauce. A tossed green salad is all you need to complete the meal.

1 tablespoon butter
1 leek (white and tender
   green), washed well and
   chopped
3 garlic cloves, minced
1 cup dry white wine
2½ pounds mussels, scrubbed
   and debearded
1 (28-ounce) can tomato puree

2 teaspoons basil
¼ teaspoon fennel seeds
¼ teaspoon crushed hot red
   pepper flakes
2 celery ribs, chopped
½ cup chopped red bell pepper
¼ teaspoon salt
¼ teaspoon pepper

1. In a 5-quart nonreactive Dutch oven, heat butter over medium-high heat until melted. Add leeks and half the garlic. Cook, stirring, until leeks are softened, 2 to 3 minutes. Add wine, cover, and heat to boiling over high heat.

2. Add mussels, cover, and return to a boil over high heat. Reduce heat to medium and steam for 4 to 6 minutes, or until shells open. With a slotted spoon, transfer mussels to a large serving bowl and keep warm; discard any unopened shells.

3. To make sauce, strain broth remaining in pan through cheesecloth to remove sand; return to pot. Cook 2 minutes over high heat. Stir in remaining garlic, tomato puree, basil, fennel seeds, hot pepper flakes, celery, red bell pepper, salt, and pepper. Heat to boiling, reduce heat to medium, and cook 5 minutes.

4. Ladle sauce into 3 or 4 large, shallow soup bowls. Divide the mussels among the bowls, placing on top of sauce. Serve with crusty bread for dipping in sauce.

45 OSSO BUCO
Prep: 15 minutes   Cook: 2½ hours   Serves: 5 to 6

This classic dish has been a favorite for decades. This version cooks away on the top of the stove for 2 hours. A squeeze of lemon juice added just before serving adds a delightful fresh flavor. Serve over pasta or with rice.

3 **pounds veal shanks**	1 **(28-ounce) can crushed**
½ **cup flour**	**tomatoes with added**
½ **teaspoon pepper**	**puree**
¼ **teaspoon paprika**	2 **celery ribs, chopped**
3 **tablespoons vegetable oil**	1 **teaspoon salt**
1 **small onion, chopped**	2 **to 3 tablespoons lemon juice**
2 **garlic cloves, minced**	
½ **cup white wine**	
4 **carrots, peeled and coarsely**	
chopped	
4 **baking potatoes, coarsely**	
chopped	

1. Dredge veal shanks in flour mixed with ¼ teaspoon pepper and paprika. Shake off excess.

2. In a 5-quart nonreactive Dutch oven, heat oil until very hot. Add shanks and cook over medium-high heat, turning, until brown all over, 10 to 15 minutes; remove to a plate.

3. Add onion and garlic to pan. Cook, stirring occasionally, until onions are soft and translucent, 2 to 3 minutes. Stir in wine, carrots, potatoes, ½ can crushed tomatoes, celery, salt, and remaining ¼ teaspoon pepper. Heat to boiling.

4. Return shanks to pan, submerging in tomato mixture. Top with remaining crushed tomatoes. Cover and heat to boiling. Reduce heat to low and simmer 2 hours, or until veal is very tender. Sprinkle with lemon juice before serving.

46   PORK RAGOUT
Prep: 15 minutes   Cook: 1¾ hours   Serves: 4 to 6

A wonderful combination for a chilly evening.

¼ cup olive oil
1½ pounds boneless pork
     shoulder, cut into 1½-inch
     cubes
¼ cup flour
1 (14½-ounce) can chicken
     broth
½ cup dry white wine
1 teaspoon tarragon
½ teaspoon paprika
1 teaspoon salt

¾ teaspoon pepper
     Grated peel of 1 orange
1 (10-ounce) basket pearl
     onions, peeled and
     trimmed
¼ pound fresh mushrooms,
     quartered
6 to 8 carrots, peeled and cut
     into 1½-inch lengths
1½ pounds red potatoes,
     scrubbed and quartered

1. Preheat oven to 350°. In a 5- or 6-quart Dutch oven, heat oil over medium-high heat until hot. Add pork cubes and cook, stirring often, 7 or 8 minutes, or until browned. Remove to a plate.

2. Add flour and cook, stirring, 1 minute. Add broth and wine and bring to a boil, whisking until thickened and smooth, 1 to 2 minutes. Add tarragon, paprika, salt, pepper, orange peel, onions, mushrooms, carrots, potatoes, and pork; mix well.

3. Cover and bake 1½ hours, until pork is tender.

47   COUNTRY RIBS WITH SAUERKRAUT
Prep: 20 minutes   Cook: 2 hours 35 minutes   Serves: 6 to 8

A cross between a soup and a stew, this is one terrific dish.

3 pounds country-style pork
     ribs
1 tablespoon garlic powder
2½ pounds russet potatoes,
     peeled and quartered
2 large onions, quartered
1 pound Polish kielbasa
     sausage, sliced ½-inch
     thick

2 (1-pound) jars sauerkraut,
     rinsed and drained
1 (1-pound) package frozen
     baby carrots
1½ teaspoons salt
½ teaspoon pepper
¾ pound Swiss chard,
     shredded

1. Place ribs in a 6-quart Dutch oven or large pot with enough water to cover. Stir in garlic powder. Cover and heat to boiling. Reduce heat to medium and cook, covered, 1½ hours. Skim foam from top.

2. Add potatoes and onions. Cover and cook over medium-low heat 45 minutes.

3. Add sausage, sauerkraut, carrots, salt, and pepper. Cook, covered, 15 minutes.

4. Stir in chard; cover and let stand 5 minutes. Serve in soup bowls.

Chapter 2

Pasta Pot

With pasta a consuming national passion, it's only natural that it should appear frequently on weeknight menus. Regardless of whether you opt for the interesting variety of fresh pastas available in the refrigerator deli sections of supermarkets (which are of excellent quality and cook in 1 to 3 minutes) or the dried variety (which take about 10), pasta lends itself fabulously to one-pot creations. The possibilities are endless, sporting any number of fresh or frozen vegetables, exotic convenient canned items, and cooked meats, fish, or poultry. Even meatless renditions are delicious.

One-pot pasta dishes are nothing new in my house. As a working mother of two, always racing against the clock to get dinner on the table, pasta is often the base for my one-dish meals. I keep several packages of fresh pasta stashed in the freezer to pull out on a moment's notice. If any recipes in this section call for fresh pasta and you only have dried on hand, by all means just substitute the dried and increase the pasta cooking time by 8 to 10 minutes.

The fastest—and easiest—way to make a one-pot pasta meal is right in the pasta cooking pot. Once cooked, simply drain off the water, leaving the pasta in the pan. Or if it's a very large pot, you may prefer to drain the pasta into a colander and return it to the pot. Specialty pasta pots allow you to lift out the pasta, leaving the water behind. If it's necessary to cook fresh vegetables for the dish, simply toss them into the pasta water the last few minutes of pasta cooking time. It saves time and avoids extra pans to clean.

Then it's simply a matter of adding the sauce ingredients—for instance, fresh or canned cut-up tomatoes, chopped fresh or dried basil, olives, cheese, artichokes, ripe olives, walnuts, shrimp, cut-up cooked chicken or smoked turkey, scallions, carrots, garlic, a little olive oil, sometimes vinegar, or whatever else strikes the fancy. Cream in combination with Dijon mustard makes a wonderful rich sauce, as does cream cheese combined with milk. For interesting color, texture, and shape, vary the pastas; try spinach pastas and even black squid ink, chili, or other flavored pastas, if available.

Depending on the combination of ingredients, sometimes I heat the mixture through until hot, while on other occasions I serve the dish at room temperature, salad style. My children are adventurous and always look forward to the next new creation. Use the recipes that follow as a source of inspiration. Tailor the ingredients to suit personal tastes and lifestyles.

And don't be afraid to experiment with what's in your refrigerator. Once you get going, you'll be amazed at the number of combinations possible.

The pasta pot is guaranteed to yield some mighty wonderful eating. Choose from tempting concoctions like Stove-Top Tuna and Noodles, Tex-Mex Chicken Pasta, Fettuccine with Basil, Turkey, and Walnuts, or Tomato and Basil Linguine. You'll never get bored.

48   DILLED TUNA FETTUCCINE
Prep: 5 minutes   Cook: 8 to 9 minutes   Serves: 4 to 5

For a stove-top tuna dish in a jiffy, try this one. Zipped up with dill weed, Dijon mustard, white wine, and bell peppers, this pasta combination makes a refreshing meal.

1 (9-ounce) package fresh
  fettuccine
1 medium red bell pepper, cut
  into 1½-inch-long thin
  strips
1 medium green bell pepper,
  cut into 1½-inch-long thin
  strips
3 scallions, chopped

1 cup dry white wine
2 garlic cloves, minced
¾ teaspoon dried dill weed
2 to 3 teaspoons Dijon
  mustard
¼ teaspoon pepper
2 (6½-ounce) cans water-
  packed solid white tuna,
  well drained

1. In a large pot of boiling salted water, cook fettuccine until just tender, 2 to 3 minutes; drain well. Return pasta to pot.

2. Stir in red and green pepper strips, scallions, ¾ cup wine, and garlic. Heat to boiling, stirring. Reduce heat to medium-low, cover, and simmer 5 minutes.

3. Stir in remaining ¼ cup white wine, dill weed, mustard, pepper, and tuna. Heat through and serve immediately.

49 QUICK MACARONI AND CHEESE WITH TUNA

Prep: 5 minutes   Cook: 10 to 15 minutes   Serves: 3 to 4

This is one of my children's favorite standby dinner entrées when time is at a premium. It beats ending up at a fast-food establishment, especially at the end of a long day.

1 (7¼-ounce) package
    macaroni and cheese
    dinner
2 tablespoons margarine or
    butter
¼ cup milk

2 tablespoons dry sherry
    (optional)
1 (6½- or 7-ounce) can tuna
    packed in water, drained
2 cups frozen peas and carrots,
    thawed

1. In a large pot, cook macaroni from package in boiling salted water according to package directions until tender, 7 to 10 minutes. Drain well.

2. Over low heat, stir in margarine, milk, sherry, and cheese sauce mix from macaroni package. Cook, over medium-high heat, stirring, 2 to 3 minutes, until well blended. Stir in tuna, vegetables, and pasta. Heat through. Serve immediately.

50 EASY TUNA PASTA

Prep: 10 minutes   Cook: 10 minutes   Serves: 4

Serve this versatile pasta dish at room temperature or chilled. Don't leave out the mustard; it's the little secret to zipping up the salad. A favorite with my son, he prefers this pasta chilled.

8 ounces small pasta shells
1 (7½-ounce) can solid white
    tuna packed in water,
    well drained
½ cucumber, peeled, seeded,
    and chopped
1 tomato, chopped
1 cup sour cream or plain
    nonfat yogurt

2 tablespoons red wine
    vinegar
2 tablespoons prepared
    yellow mustard
2 tablespoons minced fresh
    dill, or 1 tablespoon dried
    dill weed
½ teaspoon salt
¼ teaspoon pepper

1. In a large pot of boiling salted water, cook pasta just until tender, 8 to 10 minutes. Drain, then rinse with cold water and drain again. Return pasta to pot.

2. Stir in all remaining ingredients until well mixed. Serve immediately on lettuce leaves or refrigerate and serve chilled.

51 STOVE-TOP TUNA AND NOODLES
Prep: 5 minutes   Cook: 16 to 18 minutes   Serves: 3 to 4

When you want tuna noodle casserole in no time flat, opt for this stove-top version.

6 ounces egg noodles (½ of a
    12-ounce package)
1 (10¾-ounce) can condensed
    cream of asparagus or
    cream of mushroom soup
½ cup milk

¼ teaspoon garlic powder
1 (6½-ounce) can tuna packed
    in water, drained
1½ cups frozen peas and carrots,
    thawed
    Freshly ground pepper

1. In a large pot of boiling water, cook noodles until just barely tender, 8 to 10 minutes. Drain well. Return noodles to pot.

2. Stir in undiluted soup and milk; mix until well blended. Heat over medium-low heat until hot and bubbly, about 5 minutes

3. Stir in tuna, peas and carrots, and pepper. Cook, stirring, until hot throughout, about 3 minutes. Serve immediately.

52 LINGUINE WITH CLAM SAUCE
Prep: 5 minutes   Cook: 11 minutes   Serves: 4

Serve this tasty classic with a tossed green salad.

1 (8- or 9-ounce) package fresh
    linguine
3 tablespoons butter, at room
    temperature
2 large garlic cloves, crushed
    through a press
1 cup light cream or
    half-and-half
2 (6½-ounce) cans chopped
    clams, drained

⅓ cup finely chopped parsley
3 tablespoons dry sherry
2 tablespoons fresh lemon
    juice
2 teaspoons white wine
    Worcestershire sauce
¼ teaspoon pepper
    Dash of hot pepper sauce
3 tablespoons grated
    Parmesan cheese

1. In a large saucepan of boiling salted water, cook pasta just until tender, 2 to 3 minutes. Drain well.

2. Add butter and garlic to pot and cook, over medium heat, tossing, 2 to 3 minutes. Stir in cream, clams, parsley, sherry, lemon juice, Worcestershire sauce, pepper, and hot sauce. Cook over medium heat, stirring often, about 5 minutes, or until heated through. Add cheese and pasta and toss well over heat 1 minute to heat through.

LINGUINE WITH HAM

Substitute 1½ cups chopped cooked ham for clams. Stir in 1 (10-ounce) package frozen peas, thawed, along with ham.

53 FETTUCCINE WITH CREAMY MUSTARD CHICKEN SAUCE

Prep: 5 minutes   Cook: 5 to 6 minutes   Serves: 4

Pick up cooked chicken at the market to use in this creamy dish, or cook extra chicken ahead to have on hand for this.

1 (9-ounce) package fresh
    spinach fettuccine
¾ cup heavy cream
1½ to 2 tablespoons Dijon
    mustard

1½ cups shredded or diced
    cooked chicken or turkey
½ cup chopped roasted red
    pepper or pimiento

1. In a large pot of boiling salted water, cook fettuccine until just tender, 2 to 3 minutes. Drain well. Return pasta to pot.

2. Add cream and mustard to pasta in pot. Cook over medium heat, tossing, until well mixed and hot, about 2 minutes. Mix in chicken and red peppers. Heat through. Serve immediately.

54 PASTA WITH TOMATOES, BLACK OLIVES, AND CAPERS

Prep: 5 minutes   Cook: 15 minutes   Serves: 4

Capers add a special flavor to most any dish, including this one, which rated raves with tasters.

1 (8- or 9-ounce) package
    curlies or corkscrew
    noodles
2 tablespoons olive oil
2 garlic cloves, crushed
    through a press
2 medium tomatoes, chopped
1 (6-ounce) can pitted ripe
    olives, drained and cut up

3 tablespoons drained capers
2 tablespoons finely chopped
    parsley
2 tablespoons grated
    Parmesan or Romano
    cheese

1. In a large pot of boiling salted water, cook pasta until tender, about 10 minutes. Drain well. Return pasta to pot.

2. Add olive oil, garlic, tomatoes, olives, capers, and parsley. Cook over medium heat, tossing frequently, 5 minutes. Sprinkle with cheese and serve.

55 CHICKEN TEQUILA FETTUCCINE
Prep: 15 minutes   Cook: 5 to 6 minutes   Serves: 3 to 4

1 (9-ounce) package fresh spinach fettuccine
1 medium green bell pepper, cut into thin strips
1 medium red bell pepper, cut into thin strips
1 medium yellow bell pepper, cut into thin strips
1 small red onion, chopped
⅓ cup chopped cilantro

½ teaspoon minced fresh jalapeño pepper, or ⅛ teaspoon cayenne
½ teaspoon garlic salt
¼ cup tequila
⅔ cup heavy cream
2½ cups thin strips of cooked chicken or turkey
⅛ teaspoon pepper
1 lime, cut into wedges

1. In a large pot of boiling salted water, cook fettuccine until almost tender, 2 to 3 minutes; drain well.

2. Add green, red, and yellow bell peppers, red onion, cilantro, jalapeño pepper, garlic salt, tequila, and cream to pasta in pot. Heat to boiling over high heat, tossing often. Stir in chicken and pepper. Cook 2 to 3 minutes, or until bell peppers are tender and chicken is heated through.

3. Serve with lime wedges to squeeze over fettuccine before eating.

56 TEX-MEX CHICKEN PASTA
Prep: 10 minutes   Cook: 10 to 12 minutes   Serves: 6

The flavors of Mexican-style cuisine are blended in this simple dish.

8 ounces rotini or spiral twist pasta
3 tablespoons red or white wine vinegar
1 tablespoon olive oil
½ medium green bell pepper, chopped
4 scallions, chopped
1½ cups chopped fresh tomatoes, or 1 (14-ounce) can Italian peeled tomatoes, drained and chopped

1 cup canned or frozen thawed corn kernels
1 (4-ounce) can diced green chiles
1½ cups chopped cooked smoked turkey or chicken
½ teaspoon ground cumin
¾ teaspoon salt
¼ teaspoon pepper
Red lettuce leaves

1. In a large pot of boiling salted water, cook rotini until just tender, 10 to 12 minutes; drain well. Return pasta to pot.

2. Add vinegar, oil, green pepper, scallions, tomatoes, corn, green chiles, turkey, cumin, salt, and pepper. Toss until well mixed. Serve at room temperature or chilled on red lettuce leaves.

57   TOMATO AND BASIL LINGUINE
Prep: 10 minutes   Cook: 2 to 3 minutes   Serves: 6

A great dish to serve when summer tomatoes are at their best.

1 (9-ounce) package fresh linguine
1 bunch fresh broccoli, cut into ¾-inch florets
4 ripe plum tomatoes, seeded and chopped
3 tablespoons red wine vinegar

3 tablespoons olive oil
3 scallions, chopped
¼ cup chopped fresh basil
½ teaspoon salt
⅛ teaspoon pepper
Grated Parmesan cheese

1. In a large pot of boiling salted water, cook linguine and broccoli until just tender, 2 to 3 minutes; drain well. Transfer to a large bowl.

2. Add all remaining ingredients except cheese and toss with linguine and broccoli. Serve warm, at room temperature, or chilled. Pass a bowl of grated Parmesan cheese on the side.

SHRIMP, TOMATO, AND BASIL LINGUINE

Stir in ½ pound cooked, peeled, deveined medium to large shrimp, tossed with 2 tablespoons fresh lime juice, along with all remaining ingredients.

58   RAINBOW PASTA DINNER
Prep: 15 minutes   Cook: 8 to 10 minutes   Serves: 6

This easy flexible dish allows for many options. Vary the protein and dressing choices to suit personal taste.

1 (8-ounce) package rainbow spirals or curlies
⅓ cup chopped red bell pepper (½ small)
4 carrots, peeled and shredded
1 cup frozen peas, partially thawed

2 scallions, chopped
1 celery rib, chopped
1 cup diced cooked chicken, turkey, or ham
½ to ¾ cup Italian dressing
½ teaspoon salt
¼ teaspoon pepper
6 cups shredded lettuce

1. In a large pot of boiling salted water, cook pasta until just tender, 8 to 10 minutes. Drain, then rinse with cold water and drain again. Transfer to a large bowl.

2. Add all remaining ingredients except lettuce to pasta. Toss to blend well. Serve at room temperature or chilled on a bed of shredded lettuce.

59   LINGUINE GORGONZOLA
Prep: 5 minutes   Cook: 3 to 4 minutes   Serves: 4

This is a quick-fix idea. Simply add a simple salad (pick one up at a salad bar) and you can have dinner on the table pronto.

1 (9-ounce) package fresh
   linguine
1 cup crumbled Gorgonzola
   cheese (about 6 ounces)
¾ cup heavy cream

½ cup chopped roasted red
   pepper
½ cup chopped watercress
⅛ teaspoon pepper

1. In a large pot of boiling salted water, cook linguine 1 to 2 minutes, or until tender. Drain well. Return pasta to pot.

2. Over medium heat, stir in cheese and cream. Cook, stirring often, until cheese is melted, about 2 minutes.

3. Stir in red pepper, watercress, and pepper. Heat through.

60   QUICK ANGEL HAIR AND BRIE
Prep: 5 minutes   Cook: 1 to 2 minutes   Serves: 4

When there's no time to cook, toss together this dish. It's a sophisticated and divine combination of pasta with Brie cheese and sliced pimientos along with chopped fresh parsley or basil. It may just become a favorite in your repertoire.

1 (8- or 9-ounce) package fresh
   angel hair pasta (see Note)
1 cup cut-up pieces of Brie
   cheese (about ½ pound)
1 (4-ounce) jar sliced
   pimientos, drained

3 tablespoons chopped
   parsley or basil, or 1
   teaspoon dried basil

1. In a large pot of boiling salted water, cook angel hair pasta until just tender, 1 to 2 minutes; drain well. Return pasta to pot.

2. With a sharp knife, make a few cuts through the pasta in the pot to break it up a little. Stir in Brie cheese, pimientos, and parsley; toss well. The cheese will melt from the heat of the pasta. Serve immediately.

NOTE: *If fresh angel hair pasta is unavailable, use dried cappellini and cook according to package directions.*

61 FETTUCCINE WITH BASIL, TURKEY, AND WALNUTS
Prep: 10 minutes   Cook: 10 minutes   Serves: 3 to 4

Redolent with the flavors of pesto, this dish is a breeze to make on a busy work night. Use turkey ham, which is available cooked and ready to use at supermarket meat counters.

1 (9-ounce) package fresh fettuccine
¾ cup heavy cream
1¼ cups diced, cooked turkey ham
⅓ cup chopped fresh basil

1 to 2 tablespoons grated Parmesan cheese
Dash of crushed hot pepper flakes
⅓ cup chopped walnuts, toasted if desired

1. In a large pot of boiling salted water, cook noodles until almost tender, 2 to 3 minutes. Drain well.

2. Add cream, turkey ham, basil, cheese, and hot pepper flakes to pot. Cook over medium heat 5 minutes, stirring occasionally, until very hot and well blended. Add pasta and walnuts and cook, tossing, 1 to 2 minutes, until heated through. Serve immediately.

62 SPEEDY TOMATO-SAUCED PASTA WITH SPINACH
Prep: 5 minutes   Cook: 6 to 7 minutes   Serves: 6

You will be amazed at how quickly you can turn out this refreshing pasta main dish, which rates high marks with diners. It reminded my teenage daughter of a terrific dish she's fond of ordering at her favorite Italian restaurant.

1 (9-ounce) package fresh linguine
1 tablespoon olive oil
1 garlic clove, minced
1 (28-ounce) can cut-up, peeled tomatoes, undrained

2 cups chopped fresh spinach
¼ cup chopped fresh basil, or 1½ teaspoons dried
3 tablespoons drained capers
¾ teaspoon salt
¼ teaspoon pepper
Grated Parmesan cheese

1. In a large pot, cook linguine in boiling salted water until almost tender, 1 to 2 minutes. Drain well. Return pasta to pot.

2. Add all remaining ingredients to pot. Cook over medium heat, stirring often, until hot and bubbly, about 5 minutes. Serve with a generous topping of grated Parmesan cheese.

63   CREAMY DIJON PASTA WITH VEGETABLES
Prep: 5 minutes   Cook: 20 to 25 minutes   Serves: 4

If you want to make a creamy sauce for pasta in a jiffy—and all in one pot —try this recipe. Cream cheese in combination with milk is the secret. My children are partial to pasta fixed this way. And numerous variations of vegetables and meats are feasible. Try the combinations of foods your family enjoys.

6 ounces fusilli or tubular pasta
6 ounces cream cheese, at room temperature
½ cup milk
1½ to 2 tablespoons Dijon mustard
1 cup diced cooked ham or chicken

1 (16-ounce) package frozen broccoli, carrots, and cauliflower, thawed and drained
1 (4½-ounce) jar sliced mushrooms, drained
½ teaspoon salt
¼ teaspoon pepper
½ cup grated Parmesan cheese

1. In a large pot of boiling salted water, cook fusilli until just tender, 10 to 12 minutes. Drain well.

2. Add cream cheese and milk to pot. Cook over medium heat, stirring constantly, until cream cheese is melted and well blended with milk. Add pasta and toss to coat.

3. Reduce heat to medium-low. Stir in mustard, ham, vegetables, salt, and pepper. Cook, stirring occasionally, until vegetables are very hot and crisp-tender, 5 to 7 minutes. Serve topped with a sprinkling of grated Parmesan cheese.

64   BLACK PASTA WITH CALAMARI
Prep: 15 minutes   Cook: 6 to 7 minutes   Serves: 4

Squid ink pasta, which is black, can be purchased at specialty stores and some supermarkets. Calamari steaks are available frozen. The dish would also be wonderful prepared with a pound of raw, peeled, and deveined shrimp rather than calamari, if desired.

¼ cup plus 1 teaspoon olive oil
1 (12-ounce) package squid ink pasta
1 stick (¼ pound) butter
12 garlic cloves, minced

1 pound frozen calamari steaks, thawed and diced
3 tablespoons grated Parmesan cheese

1. In a large pot of boiling salted water with 1 teaspoon olive oil, cook pasta until just tender, 3 to 4 minutes, or according to package directions. Drain pasta and place in an attractive serving dish. Cover with foil and keep warm.

2. In same pan, heat remaining ¼ cup oil and butter over medium-high heat until butter is melted. Add garlic and cook until fragrant, 10 to 15 seconds. Stir in calamari and cook 1 minute. Pour over pasta; toss to combine. Sprinkle cheese over top and serve.

---

65 SPICY THAI CHICKEN PASTA
Prep: 15 minutes   Cook: 4 to 5 minutes   Serves: 6

A Thai-inspired creation. Serve at room temperature immediately after preparing or refrigerate and serve chilled. Either way, it's a delectable one-dish meal.

1 **(12-ounce) package Chinese water noodles***
¼ **cup peanut butter**
¼ **cup water**
⅓ **cup rice vinegar**
3 **tablespoons Asian sesame oil**
2 **tablespoons mild soy sauce**
1 **tablespoon hoisin sauce**
1 **to 1½ teaspoons hot chili oil**
½ **teaspoon sugar**
¼ **teaspoon garlic powder**
¼ **teaspoon ground ginger**

3 **cups shredded carrots**
4 **scallions, chopped**
1 **cucumber, peeled, seeded and chopped**
⅓ **cup thin strips red bell pepper**
2 **cups shredded cooked chicken**
Shredded lettuce, chopped tomatoes, and crispy Chinese noodles or fresh bean sprouts, as garnish

1. In a large pot of boiling water, cook noodles until tender, 3 to 4 minutes. Drain well.

2. Return pan to low heat and add peanut butter and water, mixing until well blended. Remove from heat and add rice vinegar, sesame oil, soy sauce, hoisin sauce, hot chili oil, sugar, garlic powder, and ginger, mixing until blended.

3. Stir in carrots, scallions, cucumber, red pepper, and chicken until mixed well. Add noodles and toss.

4. Serve on a bed of shredded lettuce and garnish with tomatoes and crisp noodles or bean sprouts.

* *Available in refrigerated Asian food section in supermarkets.*

66 RIGATONI AND ASPARAGUS
Prep: 10 minutes   Cook: 10 to 15 minutes   Serves: 2 to 3

When asparagus is in season, try this quick main-dish pasta prepared in a single pot. Cook the asparagus along with the pasta during the last several minutes of cooking time.

2 cups large rigatoni	1 scallion, finely chopped
½ pound thin asparagus spears, cut into 1-inch pieces	3 tablespoons chopped fresh basil, or 1 teaspoon dried
½ cup marinara sauce	¼ teaspoon salt
2 tablespoons sour cream	¼ teaspoon pepper
1 tablespoon red wine vinegar	2 tablespoons grated Parmesan cheese

1. In a large pot of boiling salted water, cook rigatoni until barely tender, 8 to 10 minutes. Add asparagus to pot for the last 3 to 4 minutes of cooking time so that asparagus comes out crisp-tender. Drain water off and run cold water over rigatoni and asparagus in pot. Drain well.

2. Add marinara sauce, sour cream, vinegar, scallions, basil, salt, and pepper to pasta and asparagus in pot. Toss to mix well. Heat through 2 to 3 minutes. Sprinkle with cheese.

67 JIFFY MACARONI AND CRAB
Prep: 10 minutes   Cook: 10 minutes   Serves: 4

This combination is offbeat, but interesting and tasty. Cooked pasta is combined with imitation crab, lettuce, and a soy–rice vinegar mixture. It's ready to eat as soon as you finish making it. If preferred, you can also serve it chilled.

1 cup small elbow macaroni	1 cup frozen peas and carrots, thawed
3 cups finely chopped iceberg lettuce	1 tablespoon sesame seeds
3 scallions, chopped	¼ cup rice vinegar
1 (2-ounce) jar chopped pimientos, drained	¼ cup soy sauce
1 cup chopped imitation crab meat, such as Sealegs	1 tablespoon Asian sesame oil
	⅛ teaspoon pepper

1. In a large pot of boiling salted water, cook macaroni until just tender, about 10 minutes. Drain off water, leaving macaroni in pot.

2. Stir in lettuce, scallions, pimientos, crab, peas and carrots, sesame seeds, vinegar, soy sauce, sesame oil, and pepper. Toss to mix well. Serve immediately or refrigerate and serve chilled.

68 PASTA WITH BROCCOLI, SUN-DRIED TOMATOES, AND BLUE CHEESE
Prep: 10 minutes   Cook: 3 to 4 minutes   Serves: 4

This pasta meal-in-a-dish is designed for blue cheese devotees. If you want to add a little meat, try slivered pieces of cooked ham, turkey, or chicken.

1 **(9-ounce) package fresh fettuccine**
2 **cups small broccoli florets**
12 **sun-dried tomatoes, halved**

⅓ **cup crumbled blue or Gorgonzola cheese**
3 **tablespoons heavy cream Freshly ground pepper**

1. In a large pot of boiling salted water, cook fettuccine and broccoli until just tender, 2 to 3 minutes. Drain well. Return pasta and broccoli to pot.

2. Add sun-dried tomatoes, blue cheese, cream, and pepper. Heat to boiling, tossing constantly. Serve immediately.

69 CURRIED PENNE WITH SHRIMP
Prep: 5 minutes   Cook: 20 to 25 minutes   Serves: 3 to 4

The inspiration for this came from a dish sampled at an Italian restaurant. Although it's a different twist on the curry theme, it works well. Vary the amount of curry to suit personal taste; use the large amount if you like spicy foods. If you prefer, you can substitute cut-up cooked chicken for the shrimp.

8 **ounces penne or other tubular pasta**
1 **cup heavy cream**
2 **to 3 teaspoons Madras curry powder**
2 **scallions, chopped**

1 **tablespoon fresh lemon juice**
½ **pound cooked medium shrimp, shelled and deveined**

1. In a large pot of boiling salted water, cook penne until tender but still firm, 10 to 12 minutes; drain well. Return pasta to pot.

2. Add cream, curry powder, and scallions. Cook over medium heat, tossing gently, 8 to 10 minutes, until thickened slightly. Stir in lemon juice and shrimp; heat through. Serve topped with a sprinkling of grated Parmesan cheese, if desired.

70   ORZO AND VEGETABLES
Prep: 15 minutes   Cook: 10 minutes   Serves: 4 to 5

1 cup orzo
4 cups cut-up broccoli florets
   (1 bunch)
½ cup coarsely chopped,
   drained, marinated
   artichoke hearts
1 (6-ounce) can ripe olives,
   drained and coarsely
   chopped
2 medium tomatoes, chopped
2 scallions, chopped
2 tablespoons olive oil
3 tablespoons red wine
   vinegar
¼ teaspoon garlic salt
¼ teaspoon pepper
1 cup diced cooked chicken
6 to 7 cups mixed salad greens

1. In a large pot of boiling salted water, cook orzo over medium-high heat 6 minutes. Add broccoli to pot and cook 4 to 5 minutes longer, until broccoli and orzo are tender. Drain well.

2. Add artichoke hearts, olives, tomatoes, scallions, oil, vinegar, garlic salt, pepper, and chicken to pot, tossing well. Serve immediately on mixed salad greens.

71   TORTELLINI SALAD
Prep: 15 minutes   Cook: 10 minutes   Serves: 5 to 6

This colorful and attractive main-dish salad is ideal to serve for a special festive luncheon or buffet.

½ pound cheese-filled
   tortellini
¼ cup olive oil, preferably
   extra-virgin
2 tablespoons red wine
   vinegar
1 garlic clove, minced
¼ cup finely chopped parsley
1 tablespoon grated Parmesan
   cheese
¼ pound thinly sliced ham or
   prosciutto, chopped
¼ pound smoked or hickory-
   barbecued turkey,
   chopped (about 1 cup)
¼ pound mozzarella or
   provolone cheese, diced
¾ cup frozen Chinese pea
   pods, thawed and
   drained
2 carrots, peeled and
   shredded
½ red bell pepper, chopped
   Lettuce leaves

1. In a large pot of boiling salted water, cook tortellini until just tender, 8 to 10 minutes. Drain well and allow to cool 5 minutes. Return pasta to pot.

2. Add oil, vinegar, garlic, parsley, and Parmesan cheese, tossing gently until well mixed.

3. Stir in ham, turkey, mozzarella cheese, pea pods, carrots, and bell pepper, tossing until well mixed. Serve immediately, or cover and refrigerate until well chilled. Serve on a bed of lettuce leaves.

72 GREEK-STYLE PASTA SALAD
Prep: 15 minutes   Cook: 10 to 12 minutes   Serves: 4 to 5

All the flavors of a Greek salad are found in this main-dish version, which also contains pasta. Add diced cooked chicken for a change of pace.

8 ounces penne or other tubular pasta
3 tablespoons extra-virgin olive oil
2 tablespoons red wine vinegar
1 medium cucumber, peeled, seeded, and chopped
1 (2.2-ounce) can sliced ripe olives, drained
3 medium tomatoes, diced
2 scallions, chopped

1½ cups frozen green beans, thawed
½ green bell pepper, chopped
2 tablespoons chopped flat-leaf parsley
2 teaspoons oregano
1 garlic clove, minced
¼ teaspoon salt
⅛ teaspoon pepper
1 cup crumbled feta cheese (4 ounces)

1. In a large pot of boiling salted water, cook penne until just tender, 10 to 12 minutes; drain well. Rinse with cold water and drain again. Return pasta to pot.

2. Add olive oil and vinegar and toss to coat. Add cucumber, olives, tomatoes, scallions, green beans, bell pepper, parsley, oregano, garlic, salt, and pepper. Toss to mix well.

3. Sprinkle feta cheese over salad. Serve chilled or at room temperature.

73 RED AND GREEN TORTELLINI SALAD
Prep: 10 minutes   Cook: 7 to 8 minutes   Serves: 4

Perfect for a summer supper, you can produce this fresh-tasting entrée salad in minutes.

1 (8-ounce) package fresh tortellini with cheese
¼ cup red wine vinegar
3 tablespoons olive oil
2 cups frozen, thawed, French-cut green beans
1 large tomato, chopped

½ red bell pepper, chopped
2 scallions, chopped
¼ cup chopped fresh basil, or 1½ tablespoons dried
¼ teaspoon salt (optional)
⅛ teaspoon pepper

1. In a large pot of boiling salted water, cook tortellini until just tender, 7 to 8 minutes. Drain well. Return pasta to pot.

2. Stir in vinegar, oil, and all remaining ingredients. Mix well. Adjust seasoning to taste. Serve immediately on assorted lettuce leaves or refrigerate and serve chilled.

NOTE: *Cut-up leftover cooked chicken, turkey, or ham can also be added to the salad, if desired.*

Chapter 3

Skillet Suppers

Start with a skillet, and there's no limit to what you can cook on top of the range. Skillets, or frying pans, are a boon to those searching for a quick dinner solution. In fact, this chapter is the largest one in the book, which isn't difficult to understand when you see how in-step these recipes are with today's one-stop, fast-paced, cooking and eating styles. Recipes like Garden Frittata, Cheese Quesadilla, Sloppy Joe Muffins, Jiffy Chicken Stew, and Italian Turkey Cutlets can be lifesavers when you're on the run and just too busy to plan dinner.

A skillet is a shallow cooking pan with flared or straight sides. Many come with a lid. For best results, the pan base should be thick and heavy to spread the heat evenly.

The large surface area on the bottom of the pan is responsible for helping to make skillet dishes so quick and easy. Unlike saucepans, a skillet exposes a larger portion of the food to heat, resulting in faster cooking time and more evaporation to thicken sauces.

Remember that a skillet should be the right size for the job. Too little food cooked in a large pan might scorch, while too much might overflow. Only two sized skillets are required for the recipes here—10 and 12 inches in diameter. For best results, use those that have nonreactive linings, so there's no chance of having a reaction with acidic foods, spinach, or wine. (The traditional American skillet made of cast iron was avoided in testing these recipes for this reason, though it is an excellent pan for nonreactive foods.) Although some food experts shy away from stainless steel skillets, favoring copper and aluminum, I've used heavy stainless steel for years without any problems, and it is my skillet material of choice.

One secret to success with skillet meals is checking on cooking progress often. Stove-top heat settings and heat outputs vary from stove to stove and are also dependent on whether the unit is gas or electric. Recipe directions are only guidelines. Common sense plays a key role in ending up with successful results.

With a little culinary ingenuity, it takes only a few minutes to transform humble chicken, steaks, ground meat, turkey slices, sausages, and fish into stylish mélanges. A number of the recipes here feature shortcuts, such as utilizing frozen vegetables, ground meats, and canned items, such as water chestnuts, olives, and mushrooms, to make chop-free, speedy suppers.

Here is a fast-paced Easy Skillet Lasagne, which is finished in just half an hour. There is a Mexican-Style Party

Chicken, Braised Halibut with Vegetables and Rice, Hot Santa Fe Chicken, Steamed Sole with Tomato, Fennel, and Orzo, Skillet Pork Chops, Italian Style, Turkey with Bananas and Peanuts, Skillet Tamale Pie, Spicy German Bratwurst, and much, much more.

The race against the clock is on—see how fast you can get dinner on the table. And have fun doing it!

74   SUPER TACO SKILLET PIE
Prep: 15 minutes   Cook: 7 to 8 minutes   Serves: 4 to 5

This is a take-off on the ever-popular taco dip, but this version with meat can serve as a main-dish entrée.

1 pound lean ground beef	½ small green bell pepper, chopped
1 medium onion, chopped	½ cup shredded cheddar cheese
1 (16-ounce) can refried beans	
1 (4-ounce) can diced green chiles	½ cup shredded Monterey Jack cheese
¼ teaspoon garlic powder	¼ to ¾ head iceberg lettuce, shredded
¾ cup sour cream	
½ teaspoon ground cumin	¾ to 1 cup crushed tortilla chips
½ teaspoon chili powder	
2 medium tomatoes, chopped	Guacamole (recipe follows)
1 (2.2-ounce) can sliced ripe olives, drained	

1. In a 10-inch skillet, cook beef and onion, stirring occasionally, over medium heat, until beef is browned, about 5 minutes. Drain off any fat.

2. Stir in refried beans, green chiles, and garlic powder. Heat to boiling, stirring occasionally. Remove from heat, scrape down sides of skillet with a spatula, and spread mixture evenly in skillet.

3. Combine sour cream with cumin and chili powder and spread on top. Place tomatoes in a circle around outer edge of sour cream. Place ripe olives in circle inside tomatoes and place green pepper in center.

4. Sprinkle top with cheeses. To serve, cut into wedges and carefully lift out. Top with lettuce, tortilla chips, and Guacamole.

GUACAMOLE

Mash 1 peeled and seeded ripe avocado with 2 tablespoons lemon juice and ¼ teaspoon garlic salt. Stir in 1 tomato, finely chopped, if desired.

75   CHUCKWAGON BEEF AND BEANS
Prep: 10 minutes   Cook: 20 to 25 minutes   Serves: 4 to 5

Buttermilk biscuits cook atop a beef and bean mixture in a skillet for a dumpling-like effect. Sprinkle them with a little grated cheddar cheese, if you like, for extra flavor.

1 **pound lean ground beef**	⅓ **cup barbecue sauce**
½ **green bell pepper, chopped**	2 **tablespoons prepared**
1 **(15½-ounce) can barbecue**	**yellow mustard**
beans, undrained	½ **cup water**
1 **(15-ounce) can Great**	1 **(7.5-ounce) can buttermilk**
Northern (large white)	**biscuits**
beans, rinsed and drained	

1. In a 10-inch skillet, cook beef over medium-high heat, stirring occasionally, until browned, 6 to 8 minutes. Drain off any fat.

2. Stir in green pepper, undrained barbecue beans, drained white beans, barbecue sauce, mustard, and water. Heat to boiling, stirring occasionally, over medium heat.

3. Cut biscuits in half and place around edge and in center of skillet. Reduce heat to medium, cover, and simmer 12 to 15 minutes, until biscuits are cooked in center (they will be like dumplings and will not brown). Serve immediately.

76   SLOPPY JOE MUFFINS
Prep: 5 minutes   Cook: 20 minutes   Serves: 4 to 5

When time is of the essence, it's faster to whip up this recipe than to drive to a fast-food restaurant.

1 **pound lean ground beef**	2 **tablespoons ketchup**
1 **green bell pepper, chopped**	1 **to 2 teaspoons**
1 **medium onion, chopped**	**Worcestershire sauce**
1 **medium zucchini, chopped**	**Salt and pepper**
1 **medium tomato, chopped**	4 **English muffins, split in**
1 **(8-ounce) can tomato sauce**	**half and toasted**

1. In a large skillet, cook beef over medium-high heat, stirring often to break up lumps, until browned, 5 to 7 minutes. Drain off excess fat.

2. Stir in green pepper, onion, zucchini, and tomato. Cook, stirring occasionally, until onion is tender, about 5 minutes. Stir in tomato sauce, ketchup, Worcestershire sauce, and salt and pepper to taste. Heat to boiling, reduce heat to low, and simmer 10 minutes.

3. Spoon mixture over muffin halves and serve open face.

77 SPANISH RICE SUPPER
Prep: 10 minutes   Cook: 40 to 45 minutes   Serves: 4 to 5

This is one of those tried-and-true weekday menu standbys that appeals to young and old alike. It's one of my son's often-requested favorites. A green salad is all that's needed to complete the meal.

1 pound lean ground beef
1 onion, chopped
½ green bell pepper, chopped
1 cup converted rice
1 (28-ounce) can cut-up, peeled tomatoes, undrained
1 (6-ounce) can tomato paste

1 cup water
2 teaspoons ground cumin
¼ cup canned diced green chiles
½ teaspoon salt
¼ teaspoon pepper

1. In a 10-inch skillet, cook beef, onion, and green pepper over medium-high heat, stirring often, until beef is browned, 8 to 10 minutes. Drain off excess fat.

2. Stir in rice, tomatoes with their liquid, tomato paste, water, cumin, and chiles. Heat to boiling, stirring occasionally. Reduce heat to low. Cover pan and simmer over low heat 30 to 35 minutes, or until rice is tender. Stir in salt and pepper. Serve immediately.

78 WINTER BEEF AND VEGETABLE MEDLEY
Prep: 15 minutes   Cook: 30 to 35 minutes   Serves: 4 to 5

This is a simple, straightforward skillet dish using the bounty of winter vegetables found in the market. Accompany with steamed brown or wild rice for an easy supper.

1 pound boneless top sirloin steak, trimmed of all fat
3 tablespoons vegetable oil
4 celery ribs, thinly sliced diagonally
5 carrots, peeled and thinly sliced diagonally
1 bunch radishes (about 10), thinly sliced
3 medium turnips, peeled, cut into quarters, and thinly sliced

½ pound fresh green beans, cut into 1½-inch pieces
2 beef bouillon cubes
¾ cup water
¼ teaspoon salt
¼ teaspoon pepper
1 tablespoon cornstarch

1. With a sharp knife, cut steak diagonally across the grain into ¼-inch slices. In a 10-inch skillet, heat 2 tablespoons oil over high heat until hot. Add beef and cook over high heat, stirring often, until beef is medium-rare, 5 to 6 minutes. Remove to a dish with any drippings.

2. Add remaining 1 tablespoon oil to skillet and heat until hot. Add celery, carrots, radishes, turnips, and green beans and cook, stirring, over medium-high heat until crisp-tender, about 5 minutes.

3. Stir in bouillon cubes, ½ cup water, salt, and pepper. Heat to boiling, stirring. Reduce heat to medium-low, cover, and cook 15 to 20 minutes, until turnips and beans are fork tender.

4. Stir in cornstarch mixed with remaining ¼ cup cold water. Heat over medium heat, stirring often, 2 to 3 minutes, until sauce clears and thickens. Return beef and drippings to skillet and heat through, stirring, 1 to 2 minutes.

---

79 MEAT LOAF OLÉ
Prep: 10 minutes   Cook: 40 to 45 minutes   Serves: 8

This stuffed beef loaf with south-of-the-border overtones makes great mealtime sandwich fare. Keep it in mind for a picnic, too.

1 (1½-pound) round loaf unsliced Sheepherder's or peasant bread
1 pound lean ground beef
1 onion, chopped
1 green bell pepper, chopped
1 (1.25-ounce) package taco seasoning mix

1 (8-ounce) can tomato sauce
1 (16-ounce) can refried beans with green chiles
1 cup shredded cheddar cheese (4 ounces)
Optional accompaniments: Shredded lettuce, guacamole, sour cream

1. Preheat oven to 350°. Slice top off bread loaf. Pull out soft inside (and reserve for another use), leaving a thick shell. Set aside.

2. In a large skillet, cook beef, onion, and green pepper over medium-high heat, stirring often, until beef is crumbly and brown, 5 to 7 minutes. Drain off excess fat.

3. Stir in taco seasoning mix, tomato sauce, and refried beans, mixing well and heating through. Stir in cheese.

4. Spoon beef filling into bread shell; replace top of loaf. Wrap tightly in foil. Bake 30 to 35 minutes, or until heated through. For ease in cutting, remove top of loaf and cut top and bottom into wedges to serve. Replace top when serving. Serve with shredded lettuce, guacamole, and sour cream alongside, if desired.

80   GROUND BEEF AND ORIENTAL VEGETABLE SKILLET SUPPER

Prep: 5 minutes   Cook: 10 to 12 minutes   Serves: 4

Whip this up in a jiffy with a little ground beef, leftover rice, and whatever vegetables you have on hand. My children love it.

½ pound ground beef or
    ground turkey
1 medium onion, chopped
1 garlic clove, crushed
    through a press
1 (14-ounce) package fresh
    cut-up chop suey
    vegetables
    (a combination of Napa or
    Chinese cabbage, bok
    choy, bean sprouts and
    celery), about 6 cups total

1½ cups cooked rice
3 tablespoons soy sauce

1. In a 10-inch skillet, cook beef over high heat, stirring often, until crumbly and browned, about 5 minutes. Drain off excess fat.

2. Stir in onion and garlic and cook 1 to 2 minutes, until onion is tender.

3. Add vegetables and stir-fry 2 to 3 minutes, or until vegetables are crisp-tender.

4. Add rice and soy sauce and cook, stirring, until heated through, about 2 minutes.

81   QUICK GREEK-STYLE SKILLET BEEF

Prep: 10 minutes   Cook: 20 minutes   Serves: 4

This is a time-saving version of a wonderful classic Greek stew. Serve over pasta or rice

1 pound boneless top sirloin
    steak, trimmed of all fat
1 tablespoon cooking oil
1 onion, halved and cut into
    thin wedges
2 garlic cloves, crushed
    through a press
1 (6-ounce) can tomato paste
½ cup dry red wine
⅓ cup water

2 tablespoons fresh lemon
    juice
⅛ teaspoon ground cumin
¼ teaspoon ground cinnamon
¾ cup crumbled feta cheese
½ cup coarsely chopped
    walnuts, toasted
3 tablespoons finely chopped
    parsley

1. With a sharp knife, cut steak diagonally across grain into thin slices. In a 10-inch skillet, heat oil over high heat until hot. Add beef and cook, stirring often, until meat loses its redness, 3 to 5 minutes. Remove meat along with any drippings to a plate.

2. Add onion and garlic to skillet and cook over medium-high heat, stirring, until onion is tender, 2 to 3 minutes. Stir in tomato paste, wine, water, lemon juice, cumin, and cinnamon. Heat to boiling, stirring. Reduce heat to low, cover, and simmer 10 minutes, stirring once or twice.

3. Return beef to skillet and heat through, 1 to 2 minutes.

4. Top with cheese and walnuts. Garnish with parsley.

82 BEEF FILLET WITH MUSHROOM-PEPPER SAUCE

Prep: 10 minutes   Cook: 15 minutes   Serves: 4

This attractive dish is a breeze to whip up on short notice for unexpected guests.

2 tablespoons butter	1 teaspoon instant beef bouillon granules
1 tablespoon olive oil	
4 (6-ounce) beef fillet steaks	½ teaspoon Beau Monde seasoning
1 bunch scallions, chopped (about 1 cup)	2 teaspoons cornstarch mixed with 1 tablespoon cold water
1 pound fresh mushrooms, sliced	
1 medium red bell pepper, cut into thin strips	Freshly ground pepper
	1 (8½-ounce) can quartered artichoke hearts, drained
1 green bell pepper, cut into thin strips	4 toasted thin bread rounds (crusts removed)
⅓ cup dry sherry	
¼ cup water	

1. In a 12-inch skillet, melt 1 tablespoon butter in olive oil over high heat. Add beef and cook, turning, until browned outside and medium to medium-rare, a total of 6 to 8 minutes, depending on thickness, or to desired doneness. Remove to a plate and keep warm. Pour any fat from pan.

2. Melt remaining 1 tablespoon butter in same skillet. Add scallions and cook, stirring, 2 to 3 minutes, until limp. Add mushrooms and peppers and cook, stirring, 3 to 4 minutes, until crisp-tender. Stir in sherry, water, bouillon, and Beau Monde seasoning; heat to boiling. Add cornstarch mixture, pepper, and artichoke hearts. Return to a boil, stirring occasionally. Cook 1 to 2 minutes, until sauce clears and thickens.

3. On each of 4 dinner plates, place beef fillet on a bread round. Top with some of sauce and serve.

83   BEEF STROGANOFF
Prep: 10 minutes   Cook: 15 minutes   Serves: 4 to 5

This dish is a classic. Serve over noodles or steamed rice.

1 pound boneless top sirloin steak	½ cup dry sherry ½ cup beef broth
2 tablespoons vegetable oil	1½ tablespoons cornstarch
2 tablespoons butter	1 cup sour cream
1 pound fresh mushrooms, sliced	1 tablespoon Dijon mustard ¼ cup chopped parsley
4 scallions, chopped	

1. Trim all excess fat from steak and cut meat diagonally across grain into thin strips. In a large skillet, heat 1 tablespoon oil over high heat. Add half of beef and cook, tossing, 2 to 3 minutes. Remove to a dish. Repeat with remaining oil and beef.

2. Add butter to skillet and, when melted, stir in mushrooms and scallions. Cook, over medium-high heat, stirring frequently, until mushrooms are tender, about 5 minutes.

3. Add sherry and boil 2 to 3 minutes to reduce slightly. Combine beef broth and cornstarch and blend well. Add to skillet and cook, stirring, until mixture boils and thickens. Stir in sour cream and mustard until blended.

4. Return beef to skillet and heat through 1 to 2 minutes, but do not boil. Garnish with chopped parsley.

CHICKEN STROGANOFF

Substitute 1 pound skinless, boneless chicken breast halves, cut into thin strips, for beef sirloin and use ½ cup chicken broth in place of beef broth.

84   BEEF AND VEGETABLES IN A PITA
Prep: 10 minutes   Cook: 8 to 11 minutes   Serves: 4 to 5

A tasty way to get a light supper on the table in a jiffy. Substitute ground turkey for ground beef, if desired.

1 pound lean ground beef	¼ teaspoon salt
1 onion, chopped	¼ teaspoon pepper
½ teaspoon minced garlic	4 to 6 pita breads, split open at one edge
½ pound fresh mushrooms, sliced	1 tomato, chopped

1¼ pounds fresh spinach,
     cleaned and chopped
	½ cup plain yogurt or sour
	     cream (optional)

2 tablespoons drained capers	

1. In a 10-inch skillet, cook beef and onion over medium-high heat, stirring often, until beef is crumbly and brown, 5 to 7 minutes. Drain off excess fat.

2. Stir in garlic, mushrooms, and spinach and cook, stirring frequently, until spinach is tender, 3 to 4 minutes. Stir in capers, salt, and pepper.

3. Spoon beef mixture into pita breads and top with chopped tomato and yogurt.

---

85   BRAISED STEAK, INDONESIAN STYLE
Prep: 10 minutes   Cook: 2¼ hours   Serves: 8

This is an adaptation of a wonderful recipe my mother shared. She serves part of it immediately after cooking, then freezes the rest of it for another meal at a future date. To make this dish even more authentic, pass condiment dishes of roasted cashews, coconut flakes, and papaya slices.

2½ to 3 pounds boneless beef round or chuck steak, trimmed of all fat	½ teaspoon ground ginger
	2 teaspoons curry powder
	1 medium onion, chopped
⅓ cup flour	½ cup mango chutney
½ teaspoon salt	⅓ cup raisins
¼ teaspoon pepper	1½ cups converted rice
2 tablespoons vegetable oil	1 (16-ounce) package frozen mixed vegetables
2 (14½-ounce) cans beef broth	
½ teaspoon garlic salt	

1. Cut meat into serving-size pieces. Mix flour, salt, and pepper together until well blended; rub mixture (with fingertips) into all sides of meat.

2. In a deep 12-inch skillet or large flameproof casserole, heat oil over high heat until hot. Add meat and cook, turning, until well browned on both sides, 8 to 10 minutes. Add 1 can of broth, garlic salt, ginger, curry powder, onion, chutney, and raisins; mix well. Heat to boiling, reduce heat to low, cover, and simmer 1½ hours.

3. Stir in remaining can of broth and rice, mixing well. Heat to boiling over high heat. Reduce heat to low, cover, and simmer 30 minutes, until rice is tender.

4. Sprinkle vegetables on top of mixture. Cover and simmer 5 to 10 minutes, or until vegetables are hot. Stir in vegetables.

86 SKILLET TAMALE PIE
Prep: 10 minutes   Cook: 45 minutes   Serves: 4 to 6

Don't turn your nose up at this dish prepared with convenient ready-made tamales until you try it. It's glorious and easily prepared comfort food that soothes the soul. Friends and family won't believe your secret when you tell them how you made it.

2 small onions, chopped
1 medium red bell pepper,
    chopped
2 medium zucchini, chopped
4 (8-ounce) packages prepared
    refrigerated beef tamales

1 cup hot water
2 cups cheddar cheese,
    shredded (½ pound)
8 cups mixed shredded lettuce
½ cup sour cream

1. Place half the onions, red pepper, and zucchini in bottom of a 12-inch skillet. Cut tamales in half lengthwise and place them, filling side up, on top of vegetables. Add hot water to skillet and top tamales with remaining onions, red pepper, and zucchini.

2. Heat to boiling, reduce heat to low, cover, and simmer 35 minutes. Sprinkle cheese. Cover and cook over low heat 5 minutes longer, or until cheese melts. Serve over greens, topped with a dollop of sour cream.

87 SKILLET MOUSSAKA SANDWICHES
Prep: 10 minutes   Cook: 20 minutes   Serves: 4 to 5

This skillet dish combines the flavors found in moussaka, but quickly, for those without much time. This tasty version, sprinkled with feta cheese, is wonderful served in pita bread. My teenage daughter found this variation most appealing and even asked for seconds.

2 tablespoons olive oil
1 pound top sirloin steak, cut
    diagonally across the
    grain into thin strips
1 garlic clove, crushed
    through a press
1 large eggplant (1½ pounds),
    peeled and cut into thin
    strips
4 scallions, chopped
½ pound fresh mushrooms,
    sliced
½ red bell pepper, cut into thin
    strips

½ green bell pepper, cut into
    thin strips
4 medium tomatoes, chopped
    (1½ cups), or 1 (14-ounce)
    can Italian peeled
    tomatoes, drained and
    chopped
2 tablespoons ketchup
2 tablespoons dry white wine
½ cup cut-up pitted ripe olives
4 or 5 (6-inch) pita breads,
    halved crosswise
4 ounces feta cheese,
    crumbled (about 1 cup)

1. In a 10-inch skillet, preferably nonstick, heat 1 tablespoon oil until very hot. Add beef and cook over medium-high heat, stirring, until meat loses its redness, about 5 minutes. With a slotted spoon, remove meat to a plate.

2. Heat remaining 1 tablespoon oil in same skillet over medium-high heat. Add garlic, eggplant, and scallions. Cook, stirring, about 5 minutes. Stir in mushrooms and red and green peppers and cook, stirring often, until peppers are crisp-tender, 4 to 5 minutes.

3. Mix in tomatoes, ketchup, white wine, and olives. Heat to boiling, reduce heat to medium-low, and simmer, uncovered, stirring frequently, 5 minutes. Stir beef into vegetable mixture and heat through.

4. Spoon meat mixture into pita bread halves and top with a sprinkling of feta cheese.

---

88 CHINESE-STYLE BEEF, BROCCOLI, AND RICE
Prep: 10 minutes   Cook: 15 minutes   Serves: 4

This recipe proves that Chinese-style cooking can be quick and easy. Be sure to cut the meat diagonally across the grain into thin slices for best results. Substitute chicken breast strips for the beef, if desired.

1¼ **pounds boneless top sirloin steak, trimmed of all fat**	1 **cup water**
½ **teaspoon ground ginger**	¾ **cup quick-cooking long-grain rice**
1 **teaspoon sugar**	1 **pound fresh broccoli,**
3 **tablespoons soy sauce**	**trimmed and cut into**
2 **teaspoons cornstarch**	**1-inch pieces**
1 **tablespoon vegetable oil**	

1. With a sharp knife, cut steak diagonally across grain into thin slices. In a medium bowl, mix together ginger, sugar, soy sauce, and cornstarch. Add meat strips and toss to mix well. Let stand 5 to 10 minutes.

2. In a 10-inch skillet, heat oil over high heat until hot. Add meat mixture. Cook, stirring over high heat, until meat loses its redness, 4 to 5 minutes. Remove to a plate.

3. Add water, rice, and broccoli to skillet and heat to boiling. Reduce heat to medium-low, cover, and simmer 5 to 6 minutes, or until broccoli is tender.

4. Return meat to skillet and heat to boiling, stirring often. Simmer, stirring, 1 minute.

CHICKEN, BROCCOLI, AND RICE

Substitute 1¼ pounds skinless, boneless chicken breast halves, cut into thin strips, for beef. Stir in ½ cup chopped red bell pepper when returning chicken to the skillet at the end of the cooking time.

89   TERIYAKI BROWN RICE AND BEEF

Prep: 20 minutes   Cook: 25 minutes   Serves: 4 to 6

Zip up roast beef with teriyaki sauce and combine with brown rice and broccoli for an interesting but easy salad.

1 (14½-ounce) can beef broth
1 teaspoon ground ginger
¼ cup fresh lemon juice
3 garlic cloves, minced
⅓ cup teriyaki thick baste and glaze sauce
½ pound fresh mushrooms, sliced
¼ teaspoon pepper
2 cups quick-cooking brown rice

1 (10-ounce) package frozen cut broccoli spears
¾ pound leftover or deli roast beef, cut into thin strips
1 pint basket cherry tomatoes
6 to 8 cups shredded romaine lettuce
3 scallions, cut into 2-inch strips

1. In a heavy 12-inch skillet or large flameproof casserole, mix together beef broth, ginger, lemon juice, garlic, teriyaki sauce, mushrooms, pepper, and brown rice.

2. Heat to boiling, stirring. Reduce heat to low, cover, and simmer 20 minutes.

3. Stir in frozen broccoli, cover, and cook 5 to 7 minutes longer.

4. Remove from heat; gently stir in roast beef and cherry tomatoes. Serve immediately on lettuce-lined plates. Garnish with scallions.

90   SAUTEED STEAK WITH BEER AND SAUERKRAUT

Prep: 15 minutes   Cook: 30 to 35 minutes   Serves: 4

Here's an easy way to make a meal reminiscent of Alsatian flavors.

1 pound boneless top sirloin steak, trimmed of all fat
2 tablespoons vegetable oil
1 medium onion, sliced
1 (12-ounce) can lager beer
1 (2-pound) jar sauerkraut, rinsed and well drained

6 small red potatoes, scrubbed and very thinly sliced
½ teaspoon caraway seeds
½ teaspoon pepper
3 cups packed chopped fresh spinach (about 8 ounces)

1. With a sharp knife, cut beef diagonally across the grain into ¼-inch slices. Cut slices in half.

2. In a 12-inch skillet, heat oil over high heat until hot. Add beef and cook, stirring, until it loses its redness, 4 to 6 minutes. Remove beef and any drippings to a plate.

3. Add onion to skillet and cook over high heat, stirring, 3 to 5 minutes, or until golden. Add beer, sauerkraut, potatoes, caraway seeds, and pepper to skillet. Stir to blend well. Heat to boiling; then reduce heat to medium-low. Cover and simmer 15 to 20 minutes, until potatoes are tender.

4. Stir in spinach, cover, and cook over medium heat 5 minutes. Return beef to skillet. Mix in and heat through, stirring 1 to 2 minutes.

91 SAVORY HAMBURGER WITH SPINACH AND RICE
Prep: 5 minutes   Cook: 35 to 40 minutes   Serves: 5 to 6

1 pound lean ground beef
1 onion, chopped
1 garlic clove, crushed
1 (28-ounce) can crushed
    tomatoes with added
    puree

1 (10-ounce) package frozen
    chopped spinach, thawed
    (do not drain)
¾ cup converted rice
1 teaspoon dried dill weed
¼ teaspoon pepper

1. In a 10-inch skillet, cook beef, onion, and garlic over medium-high heat, stirring often, until beef is crumbly and browned, about 5 minutes. Drain off excess fat.

2. Stir in tomatoes, spinach, rice, dill weed, and pepper. Heat to boiling, then reduce heat to low. Cover and simmer 30 to 35 minutes, or until rice is tender.

92 BRUNCH SCRAMBLE
Prep: 5 minutes   Cook: 15 minutes   Serves: 4

This recipe has gone by many names over the years, including Joe's Special. It's said to have originated at a San Francisco eatery. For added color, add chopped red pepper or pimiento. It's delicious with salsa stirred in or served alongside for breakfast, lunch, or supper.

1 pound lean ground beef or
    ground turkey
4 scallions, chopped
½ red bell pepper, chopped, or
    1 (2-ounce) jar sliced
    pimientos
1 (4-ounce) can mushroom
    stems and pieces, drained

1 (10-ounce) package frozen
    chopped spinach, thawed
    and drained
5 eggs
¼ teaspoon garlic salt
¼ teaspoon pepper
½ cup mild thick and chunky
    bottled salsa

1. In a 10-inch skillet, cook beef over medium-high heat, stirring occasionally, until beef browns, 5 to 7 minutes. Drain off excess fat.

2. Stir in scallions, red pepper, mushrooms, and spinach. Cook, stirring, 3 minutes.

3. Reduce heat to medium. In a bowl, beat eggs with garlic salt and pepper. Stir into skillet. Cook, stirring, until eggs are firm and cooked through, about 5 minutes. Stir in salsa or serve alongside.

93   CALF'S LIVER WITH BACON AND ONIONS
Prep: 15 minutes   Cook: 40 minutes   Serves: 4

Here's how to make liver and onions into a one-pot meal—in a skillet with red potatoes and mixed vegetables.

4 bacon slices
1 large onion, chopped
3 tablespoons flour
1 (14½-ounce) can beef broth
1 tablespoon cider vinegar
1 tablespoon Dijon mustard
¼ teaspoon salt
¼ teaspoon pepper

14 baby red potatoes (1-inch diameter), scrubbed and quartered
1 (10-ounce) package frozen mixed vegetables
1 pound calf's liver, cut into 2-inch pieces

1. In a 12-inch skillet, cook bacon over medium-high heat until crisp, about 7 minutes. Remove and set aside.

2. Add onion to bacon drippings and cook until golden, 3 to 5 minutes. Sprinkle flour over onion and cook, stirring, 1 minute. Whisk in broth and bring to a boil, whisking until mixture is thickened, 1 to 2 minutes. Add vinegar, mustard, salt, pepper, and potatoes, Stir to combine.

3. Cover and cook over medium-low heat 15 minutes, stirring once or twice to avoid sticking.

4. Stir in vegetables, then place liver pieces in gravy (pressing down into it). Cover and cook 13 to 15 minutes longer, or until liver is cooked to desired doneness. Crumble bacon and sprinkle on top.

94   APRICOT-MUSTARD CHICKEN AND BROWN RICE
Prep: 10 minutes   Cook: 40 minutes   Serves: 4

A wonderfully easy stove-top dish that is special enough to serve to company.

1 tablespoon vegetable oil
4 skinless, boneless chicken breast halves
1 medium red bell pepper, chopped
1 medium green bell pepper, chopped
4 scallions, chopped
1 (12-ounce) can apricot nectar

2 tablespoons Dijon mustard
¼ cup water
1¾ cups quick-cooking brown rice
¼ pound green beans, trimmed and cut into ½-inch pieces
½ cup chopped dried apricots

1. In a 10-inch skillet, heat oil over high heat until hot. Add chicken and cook over high heat, turning occasionally, until golden brown on both sides, 10 to 12 minutes. Remove to a plate.

2. Add red and green peppers and scallions to skillet. Cook over medium heat, stirring often, until soft, about 5 minutes.

3. Stir in apricot nectar, mustard, and water. Heat to boiling. Stir in rice, green beans, and dried apricots.

4. Return chicken to pan. Heat to boiling; reduce heat to low. Cover and cook 20 to 25 minutes, or until rice is tender.

WHITE RICE VARIATION

Proceed as recipe directs with the following changes. Increase water to ½ cup. Use 1 cup converted rice in place of brown rice. Heat to boiling, reduce heat to low, cover, and cook 25 to 30 minutes, until rice is tender.

95 JIFFY CHICKEN STEW
Prep: 10 minutes   Cook: 20 minutes   Serves: 4

When you have a hankering for stew, but time is at a premium, this should fill the bill.

4 skinless, boneless chicken breast halves
2 tablespoons vegetable oil
1 medium onion, chopped
3 celery ribs, coarsely chopped
6 carrots, peeled and thinly sliced
1 cup sliced fresh mushrooms
1 (14½-ounce) can cut-up, peeled tomatoes, undrained
⅓ cup dry white wine
½ teaspoon minced garlic
¾ teaspoon rosemary
1 teaspoon salt
⅛ teaspoon pepper
1 tablespoon quick-mixing flour
2 tablespoons cold water
1 (14½-ounce) can whole new potatoes, drained
1 (9-ounce) package frozen French-cut green beans, thawed

1. Cut chicken into ¾-inch dice.

2. In a 10- or 12-inch skillet, heat 1 tablespoon oil over high heat until hot. Add chicken and stir-fry quickly over high heat until it turns white, 3 to 4 minutes. Remove to a plate.

3. Add remaining 1 tablespoon oil to skillet and heat. Stir in onion, celery, carrots, and mushrooms. Cook over medium heat, stirring frequently, until vegetables are crisp-tender, about 5 minutes.

4. Mix in tomatoes with their liquid, white wine, garlic, rosemary, salt, and pepper. Heat to boiling. Dissolve flour in cold water and stir into stew. Heat to boiling.

5. Add potatoes and green beans. Reduce heat to medium-low and simmer 5 minutes. Mix in chicken and simmer 2 minutes longer.

96 SWEET-AND-SOUR CHICKEN AND CABBAGE

Prep: 10 minutes   Cook: 15 to 20 minutes   Serves: 5 to 6

If you like cabbage rolls, you'll enjoy the flavor of this dish, which goes together in short order in a skillet.

1 tablespoon vegetable oil	1 (16-ounce) can whole peeled
6 skinless, boneless chicken	tomatoes, undrained and
breast halves, cut into	broken up
thin strips	1 medium head green
1 medium onion, chopped	cabbage, shredded
¼ teaspoon pepper	1 cup quick-cooking long-
¼ cup white wine vinegar	grain rice
3 tablespoons brown sugar	¼ cup golden raisins
1 (15-ounce) can tomato sauce	

1. In a 12-inch skillet, heat oil over medium-high heat. Add chicken and onion to skillet and cook, stirring until chicken turns white, 4 to 6 minutes.

2. Add pepper, vinegar, brown sugar, tomato sauce, tomatoes with their liquid, cabbage, rice, and raisins. Heat to boiling, stirring, over high heat. Reduce heat to medium-low, cover, and simmer 10 minutes, or until cabbage and rice are tender.

97 MEXICAN-STYLE PARTY CHICKEN

Prep: 10 minutes   Cook: 35 to 40 minutes   Serves: 4 to 5

This dish is festive and attractive with its interesting combination of bananas, grapes, and avocado slices.

1½ tablespoons vegetable oil	1½ tablespoons chili powder
6 to 8 pieces cut-up chicken,	¼ teaspoon ground cinnamon
skinned, if desired (2½ to	½ teaspoon salt
3 pounds)	¼ teaspoon pepper
1 medium onion, chopped	3 ripe bananas, peeled and
½ red bell pepper, chopped	sliced
1 (20-ounce) can unsweetened	½ pound seedless green
pineapple chunks	grapes, cut into small
1¾ cups quick-cooking brown	bunches
rice	1 avocado, sliced

1. In a 12-inch skillet, heat oil over medium-high heat until hot. Add chicken and cook, turning, until brown on both sides and partially cooked through, 10 to 12 minutes. Remove to a plate. Drain off excess fat.

2. Add onion and red pepper to skillet. Cook, stirring often, until onion is softened, 2 to 3 minutes.

3. Drain liquid from pineapple chunks into a 2-cup measure. Add enough water to make 2 cups liquid. Add to skillet along with brown rice and pineapple chunks. Heat to boiling over high heat.

4. Mix together chili powder, cinnamon, salt, and pepper. Stir half the chili mixture into rice mixture. Place chicken on top of rice. Sprinkle chicken with remaining chili mixture. Reduce heat to low, cover, and simmer 20 to 25 minutes, until rice is tender and chicken is cooked through. Serve surrounded by bananas, grapes, and avocado slices.

98 QUICK CHICKEN CURRY
Prep: 10 minutes   Cook: 15 minutes   Serves: 4

This delicious curry becomes wonderful company fare when served with rice and assorted condiments such as chutney, unsalted peanuts, toasted coconut, raisins, chopped scallions, and pineapple chunks.

3 tablespoons butter	⅛ teaspoon thyme leaves
1 onion, chopped	½ cup chicken broth
1 large Granny Smith apple, finely chopped	½ cup dry white wine
	1 cup heavy cream
1 large garlic clove, crushed	2 teaspoons cornstarch mixed with 1 tablespoon cold water
1½ tablespoons Madras curry powder	
½ teaspoon Beau Monde seasoning	2 cups shredded cooked chicken
½ teaspoon ground cumin	

1. In a 10-inch skillet, melt butter. Add onion, apple, and garlic and cook over medium heat, stirring often, until onion is softened and translucent, about 5 minutes. Stir in curry powder, Beau Monde seasoning, cumin, and thyme. Cook over low heat, stirring occasionally, 5 minutes.

2. Stir in broth and wine and heat to boiling. Reduce heat to medium and cook about 5 minutes to reduce mixture a little. Stir in cream and heat until simmering.

3. Add cornstarch mixture and cook, stirring, until sauce thickens. Stir in chicken and heat through.

QUICK LAMB CURRY

Stir in ½ cup chopped red bell pepper in step 3. Substitute 2 cups cut-up cooked lamb (leftover from a roasted leg of lamb) for the chicken.

QUICK SHRIMP OR CRAB CURRY

Substitute 2 cups cooked, shelled, and deveined medium shrimp or 1½ to 2 cups cooked snow crabmeat for the chicken.

99 SAN JOAQUIN CHICKEN
Prep: 10 minutes   Cook: 20 to 25 minutes   Serves: 4

If you like fruits with poultry, consider this unusual dish. It's a wonderful company offering with hot cooked rice. Be sure to garnish the plate with plenty of fresh watercress or parsley sprigs.

2 tablespoons unsalted butter
1½ pounds skinless, boneless
    chicken breast halves
1 (15-ounce) can mandarin
    orange segments
¼ cup chicken broth or water
3 tablespoons red wine
    vinegar

1 tablespoon cornstarch
1 tablespoon cold water
¼ cup maraschino cherry
    syrup
½ cup maraschino cherries
½ cup dark or golden raisins

1. In a 10-inch skillet, melt butter over medium-high heat. Add chicken breasts and cook, turning once, until golden outside and white throughout, a total of 10 to 12 minutes. Remove to a plate.

2. In same skillet, heat syrup drained from oranges with broth and vinegar until boiling. Remove from heat. Whisk in cornstarch blended with cold water until well blended. Return to heat and heat to boiling, stirring constantly, until smooth and thickened.

3. Add cherry syrup, cherries, and raisins to sauce; reduce heat to low and simmer 5 minutes. Gently stir in oranges and heat a minute more. Serve chicken over hot cooked rice and top with sauce.

100 TROPICAL CHICKEN WITH FRUIT SAUCE
Prep: 10 minutes   Cook: 6 to 8 minutes   Serves: 4

For a change of pace, serve chicken with this easy spiced applesauce-based sauce dotted with pineapple pieces, banana slices, and fresh grape halves. For added color, stir in strawberry halves or other fruits in season.

4 tablespoons butter
6 skinless, boneless chicken
    breast halves
¼ to ½ teaspoon garlic powder
2 tablespoons flour
1 cup chunky applesauce
1 (8-ounce) can unsweetened
    pineapple chunks, cut in
    half, juice reserved

1 large banana, sliced
¾ cup seedless green or red
    grapes, halved
½ cup strawberry halves
2 tablespoons brown sugar
1 teaspoon ground cinnamon
    Hot cooked brown rice
    Chopped fresh watercress,
    for garnish

1. In a 10-inch skillet, melt 2 tablespoons butter over medium-high heat until hot. Add chicken, sprinkle with garlic powder, and cook until golden, 3 to 4 minutes per side. Remove to a plate.

2. In same skillet, melt remaining 2 tablespoons butter over medium heat. Stir in flour until well blended. Cook, stirring, 1 minute.

3. Stir in applesauce, halved pineapple chunks, reserved pineapple juice, banana slices, grapes, strawberries, brown sugar, and cinnamon. Heat to boiling, stirring constantly. Reduce heat and cook for 1 to 2 minutes, until slightly thickened.

4. Serve chicken over hot cooked brown rice and spoon sauce over all. Sprinkle with watercress.

---

101 CHICKEN A LA KING
Prep: 15 minutes   Cook: 20 minutes   Serves: 4

Modernize the classic standby by sautéing chicken breast tenders and saucing them with a creamy vegetable mixture. This version tastes great over toast or rice.

2 tablespoons butter	1 medium red bell pepper, chopped
1 pound skinless chicken breast tenders	½ pound fresh mushrooms, sliced
½ to ¾ pound fresh asparagus, cut diagonally into ¾-inch pieces	¼ cup dry sherry
2 tablespoons vegetable oil	¾ cup chicken broth
1 leek (white and tender green), washed well and chopped	2 teaspoons cornstarch
1 medium green bell pepper, chopped	¾ cup heavy cream
	½ teaspoon salt
	¼ teaspoon pepper

1. In a 10-inch skillet, melt butter over medium-high heat. Add chicken tenders and cook, turning occasionally, until golden brown on both sides, 5 to 7 minutes. Remove to a dish.

2. Add asparagus to drippings in skillet. Cook over medium-high heat, stirring often, until crisp-tender, about 2 minutes. Remove to dish with chicken.

3. Add oil to pan and heat over high heat until hot. Add leeks, green and red peppers, and mushrooms and cook, stirring often, until peppers are crisp-tender, about 3 minutes.

4. Stir in sherry and chicken broth. Boil, stirring occasionally, about 4 minutes, to reduce liquid slightly.

5. Mix together cornstarch and cream until smooth. Stir into skillet. Bring to a boil over high heat. Reduce heat to medium and cook, stirring, until sauce thickens, 1 to 2 minutes. Season with salt and pepper. Return chicken and asparagus to skillet and heat through, about 1 minute.

102   EASY CHICKEN AND RICE
Prep: 5 minutes   Cook: 35 minutes   Serves: 4

1 cup converted rice
1 (10¾-ounce) can condensed
   cream of chicken soup
⅓ cup dry sherry
⅔ cup water
1 (16-ounce) package frozen
   Italian-style vegetables

4 skinless, boneless chicken
   breast halves
8 drops of Worcestershire
   sauce
   Paprika

1. In a large skillet, combine rice, soup, sherry, water, and frozen vegetables; mix well. Heat to boiling, stirring.

2. Arrange chicken breasts on top of rice mixture. Sprinkle each chicken breast with a couple of drops of Worcestershire sauce. Spread with back of spoon; sprinkle with paprika.

3. Heat to boiling, reduce heat to medium, cover, and simmer 15 minutes. Remove cover and stir rice mixture under and around chicken. Reduce heat to low and continue cooking, covered, 15 to 20 minutes, or until rice is tender.

103   CHICKEN SCALLOPINI WITH MUSHROOMS AND VEGETABLES
Prep: 15 minutes   Cook: 20 minutes   Serves: 4

This dish, based on the flavors of a classic veal recipe, is a cinch to prepare. Serve with plenty of hot cooked rice and a tossed green salad.

6 skinless, boneless chicken
   breast halves
3 tablespoons vegetable oil
1 onion, thinly sliced
½ pound fresh mushrooms,
   sliced
4 carrots, peeled and chopped
2 medium zucchini, cut into
   thin strips
1 garlic clove, minced

1 large tomato, peeled and
   diced
¾ teaspoon salt
¼ teaspoon pepper
¼ teaspoon rosemary
½ cup sauterne
1 tablespoon lemon juice
3 cups hot cooked rice
¼ cup chopped parsley

1. Pound chicken breasts between sheets of wax paper until flattened evenly to about ¼ inch thickness. In a 12-inch skillet, heat 2 tablespoons oil until hot over medium-high heat. Add chicken and cook, turning until chicken is golden and cooked through, 7 to 8 minutes total. Remove to a plate.

2. Heat remaining 1 tablespoon oil in same skillet until hot. Add onion, mushrooms, carrots, zucchini, and garlic. Cook over medium-high heat, stirring often, about 5 minutes, or until onion is soft. Add tomato, salt, pepper, rosemary, sauterne, and lemon juice. Heat to boiling, reduce heat to medium-low, and simmer, uncovered, 5 minutes.

3. Return chicken to skillet. Cook 2 to 3 minutes, until heated through. Serve on a bed of hot cooked rice and garnish with chopped parsley.

104 CHICKEN AND VEGETABLES WITH BALSAMIC VINEGAR

Prep: 10 minutes   Cook: 25 to 30 minutes   Serves: 4

If you've never tried chicken with vinegar, you're in for a tasty surprise. There's something wonderfully pleasing about the combination. In this recipe, balsamic vinegar, which comes from Italy (and is available in many supermarkets, gourmet shops, or Italian specialty markets) is teamed with an assortment of vegetables including leeks, red potatoes, carrots, and bell peppers.

1 tablespoon butter	5 carrots, peeled and cut into 2-inch-long thin strips
6 skinless, boneless chicken breast halves	½ red bell pepper, cut into thin strips
1 pound baby red potatoes, sliced into thirds	¼ teaspoon garlic powder
3 shallots, chopped	½ teaspoon salt
½ cup beef broth	¼ teaspoon pepper
2 leeks (white and tender green), well washed and cut into 2-inch-long thin strips	¼ cup balsamic vinegar

1. In a 12-inch skillet, melt butter over medium-high heat. Add chicken and cook, turning, until golden brown outside and white throughout, 8 to 10 minutes. Remove to a plate.

2. Add potatoes and shallots to skillet and cook, stirring often, 2 to 3 minutes, until shallots are soft and fragrant.

3. Stir in broth, scraping and loosening brown bits on bottom of pan. Add leeks, carrots, and red peppers. Heat to boiling. Reduce heat to medium-low, cover, and simmer about 8 minutes, until potatoes are tender.

4. Stir in garlic powder, salt, pepper, and balsamic vinegar. Heat to boiling. Return chicken to pan, spoon sauce over, and cook over low heat 2 to 3 minutes to heat through.

105 ONE, TWO, THREE CHICKEN SUPPER
Prep: 5 minutes   Cook: 25 to 30 minutes   Serves: 4

When you're in a hurry to get a chicken dish on the table, this recipe should fit the bill. Serve over hot rice or top with crunchy chow mein noodles.

6 tablespoons butter	1 (16-ounce) package mixed
1 pound skinless, boneless	frozen vegetables
chicken breast halves	(cauliflower, carrots, and
1 (16-ounce) package frozen	broccoli)
French-cut green beans	½ teaspoon hot pepper sauce

1. In a 10- or 12-inch skillet, melt 2 tablespoons butter over medium-high heat. Add chicken and cook, turning, until golden on both sides and white throughout, 8 to 10 minutes. Remove to a plate.

2. Add vegetables to pan. Cover, reduce heat to medium, and steam 10 to 15 minutes, or until thawed and hot.

3. Add remaining 4 tablespoons butter to skillet along with hot sauce. Cook, stirring often, until melted and hot, about 2 minutes. Return chicken to pan and heat through.

106 CHICKEN BREASTS WITH LIME CURRY SAUCE
Prep: 5 minutes   Cook: 15 to 20 minutes   Serves: 4

This curry is speedy to prepare, but is special enough to serve to company, with its embellishments of chopped fresh tomatoes and lime slices. Pass condiments, such as chutney, raisins, and cashews.

4 tablespoons butter	2 tablespoons fresh lime juice
6 skinless, boneless chicken	2 cups light cream or half-and-
breast halves	half
½ teaspoon garlic powder	½ cup flaked coconut
½ cup chopped onion	(unsweetened, if
1½ tablespoons Madras curry	available)
powder	1½ cups chopped, seeded
1 teaspoon salt	tomatoes
¼ teaspoon pepper	Lime slices, for garnish
1 tablespoon flour	

1. In a 10- or 12-inch skillet, melt 2 tablespoons butter over medium-high heat. Add chicken, sprinkle with garlic powder, and cook, turning once, until golden, 3 to 4 minutes per side. Remove to a plate and set aside.

2. In same skillet, melt remaining 2 tablespoons butter. Add onion, curry powder, salt, and pepper. Cook, stirring, 3 minutes, or until onions are tender. Stir in flour; cook, stirring, 1 minute.

3. Stir in lime juice and light cream. Heat to boiling, stirring occasionally. Reduce heat to low and simmer 7 to 8 minutes, or until sauce has thickened. Remove from heat and stir in coconut.

4. Spoon sauce over chicken breasts and top with a sprinkling of tomatoes and lime slices. Served with hot cooked rice and assorted condiments.

---

107   HOT SANTA FE CHICKEN
Prep: 15 minutes   Cook: 30 minutes   Serves: 6

This hot brown rice mélange is seasoned with jalapeños and chili powder.

2 skinless, boneless chicken breast halves, cubed
1⅛ teaspoons salt
⅛ teaspoon pepper
2 tablespoons vegetable oil
½ cup chopped onion
1½ cups chicken broth
2 cups uncooked quick-cooking brown rice
1 (10-ounce) package frozen corn kernels, thawed

1 (15-ounce) can pinto beans, rinsed and drained
¼ cup chopped scallions
¼ cup chopped fresh cilantro
2 jalapeño peppers, seeded and minced
2 teaspoons chili powder
¼ cup balsamic or red wine vinegar
1 (10-ounce) bag corn chips

1. Season chicken breasts with ⅛ teaspoon each salt and pepper. In a 10-inch skillet, heat oil over high heat. Add chicken and cook, stirring often, until golden brown, about 5 minutes. Remove to a dish.

2. In same skillet, cook onion over medium-high heat 2 to 3 minutes, until just soft. Add chicken broth and rice to skillet. Heat to boiling over high heat. Stir and reduce heat to low. Cover and simmer until all liquid is absorbed and rice is cooked, 18 to 20 minutes.

3. Stir in corn and pinto beans. Simmer, covered, 5 minutes. Remove from heat.

4. Stir in chicken, scallions, cilantro, jalapeño peppers, chili powder, vinegar, and remaining 1 teaspoon salt. Serve immediately with corn chips alongside.

108 PEANUTTY CHICKEN AND VEGETABLES
Prep: 10 minutes   Cook: 40 minutes   Serves: 4 to 5

Peanut butter lovers will delight in this dinner-in-a-dish. It's finger-licking good.

2 tablespoons vegetable oil	1 red bell pepper, cut into 1-inch-long thin strips
1 (3-pound) broiler-fryer chicken, cut up	⅓ cup peanut butter
1 teaspoon paprika	1 cup chicken broth
2 medium onions, chopped	3 to 4 drops hot pepper sauce
4 carrots, peeled and cut into 1-inch-long thin strips	¼ teaspoon salt
1 zucchini, cut into 1-inch-long thin strips	¼ teaspoon pepper
	½ cup chopped peanuts, for garnish

1. In a deep 12-inch skillet or flameproof casserole, heat oil over medium-high heat until very hot. Add chicken, sprinkle with paprika, and cook, turning occasionally, until well-browned on both sides and cooked through, about 25 minutes. Remove chicken to a plate.

2. Drain off all except 2 tablespoons drippings from skillet. Add vegetables to skillet. Cook, stirring, until onion is tender, about 5 minutes.

3. Stir in peanut butter, broth, hot sauce, salt, and pepper. Heat to boiling, stirring until smooth. Reduce heat and simmer 5 minutes. Return chicken to pan and simmer 4 to 5 minutes, until heated through. Serve chicken over hot cooked rice. Top with sauce and sprinkle with chopped peanuts.

109 SAUTEED CHICKEN STRIPS WITH BROCCOLI AND CAULIFLOWER
Prep: 10 minutes   Cook: 20 minutes   Serves: 4 to 5

A simple dish that allows cooks to get dinner on the table fast. Serve over hot cooked rice.

3 tablespoons vegetable oil	1 chicken bouillon cube
1 pound skinless, boneless chicken breast halves, cut into thin strips	3 tablespoons dry sherry
	2 tablespoons soy sauce
6 scallions, chopped	¼ teaspoon pepper
1 pound fresh broccoli, cut into 1-inch pieces	1½ tablespoons cornstarch
	1¼ cups water
1 small cauliflower, cut into thin pieces	

1. In a 10- or 12-inch skillet, heat 2 tablespoons oil over high heat. Add chicken and cook, stirring, until cooked through, 4 to 5 minutes. Remove chicken with any drippings to a plate.

2. In same skillet, heat remaining 1 tablespoon oil over medium-high heat. Add scallions, broccoli, and cauliflower. Cook, stirring, 5 minutes. Mix in bouillon cube, sherry, soy sauce, and pepper. Combine cornstarch and water and stir in until well blended. Heat to boiling, stirring constantly, until sauce thickens. Reduce heat to low, cover, and simmer 5 to 8 minutes, until vegetables are crisp-tender.

3. Return chicken to skillet, cover, and heat through 1 minute.

110 SKILLET CHICKEN WITH COUSCOUS
Prep: 15 minutes   Cook: 45 to 50 minutes   Serves: 4 to 5

Couscous is a tiny grained semolina pasta that's used often in North African cooking. Available in supermarkets or health food stores, it adds interesting texture and dimension to this skillet creation.

2 tablespoons vegetable oil	1 cup couscous
4 chicken thighs, skinned	1 (15-ounce) can garbanzo
4 chicken drumsticks,	beans (chick-peas), rinsed
skinned	and drained
1 large onion, chopped	1 (8½-ounce) can quartered
4 carrots, peeled and thinly	artichoke hearts, drained
sliced	and diced
3 celery ribs, sliced	2 tablespoons lime juice
2 garlic cloves, minced	¼ teaspoon pepper
2 cups water	

1. In a 12-inch skillet or large flameproof casserole, heat oil over high heat until hot. Add chicken and cook, turning, until browned on both sides, 10 to 12 minutes. Reduce heat to medium-low, cover, and cook chicken 10 minutes. Remove chicken to a dish and drain off all fat and liquid from pan.

2. Add onion, carrots, and celery to skillet. Cook over medium-high heat, stirring, until onion is softened, 2 to 3 minutes. Stir in garlic, water, couscous, garbanzo beans, artichoke hearts, lime juice, and pepper. Heat to boiling, then reduce heat to medium-low. Place chicken on top of couscous mixture. Cover and cook 20 to 25 minutes, or until chicken is very tender and cooked through.

111   SWEET-AND-SOUR CHICKEN LIVERS
Prep: 15 minutes   Cook: 17 minutes   Serves: 4 to 6

Here's an innovative and tasty way to prepare chicken livers in a single dish, using a packaged frozen pasta salad mixture.

1 **pound chicken livers**
¼ **cup cornstarch**
2 **tablespoons peanut oil**
1 **medium red bell pepper, chopped**
2 **garlic cloves, mashed**
1 **teaspoon grated fresh ginger**
3 **tablespoons soy sauce**
3 **tablespoons sugar**
3 **tablespoons dry sherry**
3 **tablespoons cider vinegar**

1 **(1-pound) package frozen pasta salad Orientale (a combination of Chinese noodles, broccoli, Chinese pea pods, water chestnuts, and red bell pepper)**
1 **(20-ounce) can unsweetened pineapple chunks, drained**
6 **scallions, cut into thin 2-inch-long strips**

1. Cut livers in half and pat dry with paper towels. Shake in a plastic bag with cornstarch.

2. In a 12-inch skillet, heat oil over high heat until hot. Add red pepper and cook, stirring, 1 minute. Add livers and cook, stirring often, until brown outside but still rosy inside, about 3 minutes.

3. Add garlic and ginger and reduce heat to medium. Mix together soy sauce, sugar, sherry, and vinegar. Add to skillet, cover, and cook 8 minutes.

4. Stir in frozen pasta salad and drained pineapple chunks. Cover and cook 5 minutes longer. Garnish with scallions.

112   TURKEY SANTA FE
Prep: 10 minutes   Cook: 15 minutes   Serves: 4 to 5

Chicken breast can also be used in this recipe instead of turkey.

1 **pound boneless turkey breast tenderloins**
2 **tablespoons vegetable oil**
1 **(12-ounce) jar mild green chile salsa**
1 **cup cooked or canned black beans, drained**
1 **cup frozen corn kernels, thawed**

1 **large tomato, chopped**
2 **tablespoons chopped fresh cilantro or parsley**
1 **to 1¼ cups shredded cheddar cheese (4 to 5 ounces)**
¾ **cup corn chips**
1 **avocado, sliced**
½ **cup sour cream**

1. Remove tendons from centers of turkey tenderloins, if necessary. Cut turkey across grain into thin slices. In a large skillet, heat 1 tablespoon oil until very hot. Add half the turkey slices and cook, stirring, over high heat until no longer pink, about 5 minutes. Remove turkey to a plate. Repeat with remaining turkey slices and remaining 1 tablespoon oil. Drain off any excess fat, leaving last batch of turkey in pan.

2. Return first batch of cooked turkey to pan. Stir in salsa, black beans, corn, and tomato. Heat to boiling quickly, stirring often. Stir in cilantro. Reduce heat to medium-low and simmer 3 minutes.

3. Spoon hot turkey mixture into center of 4 or 5 dinner plates. Top each with ¼ cup shredded cheese, a sprinkling of corn chips, avocado slices, and a dollop of sour cream.

---

113 TURKEY TOSTADAS
Prep: 5 minutes   Cook: 15 to 20 minutes   Serves: 4

When time is of the essence, turn to this recipe, one used often at my house. There are several possible variations on the theme, including using leftover cooked meats and poultry instead of the ground turkey or ground beef.

1 **pound ground turkey or lean ground beef**	1 **head iceberg lettuce, shredded**
½ **cup chopped onion**	1½ **cups shredded mozzarella and/or Monterey Jack cheese**
1¼ **teaspoons ground cumin**	
¼ **teaspoon chili powder**	
1 **(4-ounce) can diced green chiles**	2 **medium tomatoes, chopped**
2 **(8-ounce) cans or 1 (15-ounce) can tomato sauce**	½ **to ¾ cup guacamole**
	Bottled or homemade salsa
4 **large corn or flour tortillas, warmed**	

1. In a 10-inch skillet, cook turkey and onion over medium-high heat, stirring often, until meat is no longer pink and onion is softened, 5 to 7 minutes. (If using ground beef, drain off any fat.)

2. Stir in cumin, chili powder, green chilies, and tomato sauce. Heat to boiling, reduce heat, and continue to cook, stirring occasionally, 10 minutes.

3. Place 1 tortilla on each of 4 serving plates. Top with turkey mixture, dividing evenly. Sprinkle each plate with lettuce, cheese, and tomatoes. Top with guacamole. Pass salsa separately. Serve with additional warmed tortillas, if desired.

NOTE: *If using leftover chopped cooked meat, heat together spices and tomato sauce and simmer 10 minutes. Then add chopped cooked meat and heat through. Proceed to make tostadas as directed.*

114   TURKEY WITH BANANAS AND PEANUTS
Prep: 20 minutes   Cook: 15 minutes   Serves: 4 to 6

You'll be amazed at how easily a rice and pasta mix can be jazzed up and turned into a really special meal-in-a-dish when you try this idea.

2 tablespoons peanut oil
1 medium onion, chopped
1 medium red bell pepper, halved and cut crosswise into thin strips
1 medium carrot, peeled and cut into thin strips
1 (4.5-ounce) package broccoli au gratin rice and pasta mix (such as Rice-A-Roni)
1 pound raw turkey breast, cut into thin strips

1 (14½-ounce) can chicken broth
1 teaspoon curry powder
½ teaspoon pepper
1 (9- or 10-ounce) package frozen broccoli cut spears
2 bananas, peeled and diced
½ cup dry-roasted peanuts
3 scallions, cut into thin 2-inch-long strips

1. In a 10-inch skillet, heat oil over medium-high heat. Add onion, red pepper, and carrot and cook, stirring often, 3 to 4 minutes, until onion is limp.

2. Add contents of rice and pasta mix, including seasonings, turkey, broth, curry powder, pepper, and broccoli. Stir to combine. Heat to boiling, reduce heat to medium-low, cover, and simmer 10 minutes. Stir in bananas and peanuts and serve, garnishing each portion with a sprinkling of scallions.

115   TURKEY WITH CRANBERRIES AND ORANGE SAUCE
Prep: 15 minutes   Cook: 30 to 40 minutes   Serves: 4 to 6

Savor all the traditional flavors of Thanksgiving in this grand-tasting dish. It's wonderful any time of the year as well when you have a hankering for a traditional meal. Next time you're having only a small gathering at Thanksgiving, consider serving this dish.

2 cups orange juice
Grated juice and zest of 1 orange
3 tablespoons orange marmalade
2 large celery ribs, sliced
1 cup fresh or frozen cranberries, washed
1 (9-ounce) package brown and white Texmati rice blend with wild rice

½ teaspoon salt
¼ teaspoon white pepper
1 pound raw turkey breast slices or cutlets, cut into thin strips
1 (9-ounce) package frozen French-style green beans
¾ cup pecan halves
¼ cup chopped parsley

1. In a 12-inch skillet, combine all the orange juice, the orange zest, orange marmalade, celery, and cranberries. Heat to boiling over high heat. Reduce heat to low.

2. Stir in rice, salt, pepper, and turkey. Cover and simmer 15 to 20 minutes, or until turkey and rice are almost cooked.

3. Add frozen green beans in ring around outside edge of pan. Sprinkle pecans in center of turkey-rice mixture. Cover and cook over medium-low heat 10 to 15 minutes longer, until beans are hot. Garnish with parsley.

116   TURKEY LETTUCE WRAP-UPS
Prep: 10 minutes   Cook: 10 to 15 minutes   Serves: 4 to 5

Wrap a tasty ground turkey mixture in lettuce leaves for a festive and fun meal. Another time serve the turkey mixture on a mound of shredded lettuce and top with peanuts.

1 **pound ground turkey**	3 **tablespoons soy sauce**
4 **scallions, sliced**	1 **teaspoon Asian sesame oil**
2 **large garlic cloves, crushed through a press**	½ **teaspoon ground ginger**
	¼ **teaspoon pepper**
¼ **pound fresh mushrooms, chopped**	2 **teaspoons cornstarch**
	½ **cup chicken broth**
1 **(8-ounce) can sliced water chestnuts, drained and chopped**	3 **tablespoons hoisin sauce (optional)**
	1 **head of lettuce, separated into leaves**
4 **carrots, peeled and shredded**	⅓ **cup chopped dry-roasted peanuts**
3 **tablespoons dry sherry**	

1. In a large skillet, cook turkey, scallions, and garlic, stirring often to break up large chunks, until turkey is no longer pink, 5 to 7 minutes.

2. Add mushrooms, water chestnuts, and carrots. Cook, stirring often, until mushrooms are just tender, 3 to 4 minutes.

3. Add sherry, soy sauce, sesame oil, ginger, and pepper. Stir together cornstarch and chicken broth until blended. Stir into skillet. Heat, stirring constantly, until sauce boils and thickens.

4. To serve, spread a little hoisin sauce, if desired, on a lettuce leaf. Spoon turkey mixture onto lettuce leaf, sprinkle with a few peanuts, roll up, and eat.

117   ITALIAN TURKEY CUTLETS
Prep: 5 minutes   Cook: 10 to 15 minutes   Serves: 4

This is a quick-fix dinner idea. If you don't have time to shred the zucchini, simply omit it and serve the dish with your choice of cooked vegetables.

2 tablespoons olive oil	½ teaspoon garlic powder
1 pound turkey cutlets	1 (8-ounce) can tomato sauce
4 medium zucchini, shredded	4 slices mozzarella cheese
4 scallions, chopped	¾ teaspoon basil

1. In a 10-inch skillet, heat 1 tablespoon oil until hot. Add half the turkey cutlets and cook over medium-high heat, turning once, until browned, 2 to 3 minutes. Remove to a plate. Repeat with remaining turkey.

2. Heat remaining 1 tablespoon oil in skillet. Add zucchini and scallions and cook, stirring, until zucchini is tender and most of the moisture has cooked off, 3 to 5 minutes. Spread zucchini mixture out evenly over surface of pan. Sprinkle with ¼ teaspoon garlic powder and drizzle half the tomato sauce evenly over zucchini.

3. Arrange turkey cutlets on top and sprinkle with remaining ¼ teaspoon garlic powder. Spoon a little tomato sauce over turkey. Place cheese slices on top of cutlets and drizzle on remaining tomato sauce. Sprinkle with basil.

4. Heat to boiling, reduce heat to medium-low, and simmer until cheese melts and turkey is tender, 5 to 7 minutes.

---

118   TURKEY-VEGETABLE BULGUR
Prep: 10 minutes   Cook: 20 minutes   Serves: 4 to 5

Bulgur wheat adds interesting texture and flavor to this easy dish.

1 pound ground turkey	2 medium tomatoes, coarsely
1 onion, chopped	chopped
1 teaspoon minced garlic	½ cup water
¼ pound fresh mushrooms,	½ cup bulgur
chopped	1 teaspoon dried Italian herbs
3 carrots, peeled and thinly	¾ teaspoon ground cumin
sliced	¼ teaspoon pepper
2 cups broccoli florets	

1. In a 10-inch skillet, cook turkey, onion, and garlic over medium heat, stirring occasionally to break up meat, until turkey has lost all trace of pink, about 7 minutes.

2. Stir in mushrooms, carrots, broccoli, and tomatoes. Cook 3 minutes.

3. Stir in water, bulgur, Italian herbs, cumin, and pepper. Heat to boiling. Reduce heat to medium, cover, and cook about 10 minutes, until bulgur is tender.

119 SKILLET PORK CHOPS AND RICE
Prep: 5 minutes   Cook: 50 minutes   Serves: 4

Fix and forget this dish, based on a package of wild and white rice mix. While it's cooking, relax a few minutes, before making a salad to accompany it. Serve with condiments of shredded coconut, peanuts, and chutney.

4 (½-inch-thick) pork loin chops, fat trimmed	1 (14½-ounce) can whole peeled tomatoes, undrained and broken up
1 (6-ounce) package long-grain and wild rice mix	4 scallions, sliced
1⅓ cups water	⅓ cup seedless golden raisins

1. In a large skillet, cook pork chops over medium-high heat, turning once, until browned on both sides, about 5 minutes. Remove to a plate.

2. Add rice and seasonings from rice mix to skillet along with water, tomatoes and their liquid, scallions, and raisins; mix well. Heat to boiling. Reduce heat to low and place pork chops on top of rice. Cover and simmer 45 minutes.

120 PORK WITH YAMS, BOK CHOY, AND RICE
Prep: 10 minutes   Cook: 40 to 45 minutes   Serves: 4 to 5

If you like yams, you'll enjoy this tasty and somewhat novel dish combining them with pork strips, bok choy, and rice in a hoisin-flavored mixture. Bok choy, also known as Chinese chard, has white stalks and green leaves at the top.

1 tablespoon vegetable oil	¾ cup converted rice
¾ to 1 pound lean boneless pork, trimmed of excess fat and thinly sliced into strips	2 cups water
	6 cups ¾-inch cubes of peeled yams (about 2 medium-large)
3 scallions, sliced	3 tablespoons dry sherry
2 cups 1-inch pieces of bok choy (about ½ pound) or cabbage	2 tablespoons hoisin sauce
	1 garlic clove, minced
	½ teaspoon ground ginger

1. In a 10- or 12-inch skillet, heat oil until hot. Add pork and stir-fry over medium-high heat until pork is lightly browned, about 5 minutes. Add scallions and bok choy and cook, stirring, over high heat 2 minutes.

2. Stir in rice and water and heat to boiling. Stir in yams, sherry, hoisin sauce, garlic, and ginger and return to a boil. Reduce heat to low, cover, and simmer 30 to 35 minutes, until yams and rice are tender.

121   SKILLET PORK CHOPS, ITALIAN STYLE

Prep: 10 minutes   Cook: 40 minutes   Serves: 4 to 5

When you want to serve pork chops in a one-dish meal, this recipe with its universally appealing Italian flavor, is a good choice.

1 tablespoon vegetable oil	¾ cup converted rice
6 center-cut pork chops, cut ½-inch thick	½ cup chopped green bell pepper
½ teaspoon salt	1 (9-ounce) package frozen Italian green beans, partially thawed
¼ teaspoon pepper	
1 (15-ounce) can tomato sauce	
2 garlic cloves, minced	6 thin slices mozzarella cheese
1½ teaspoons basil	2 tablespoons grated Parmesan cheese
1½ cups water	

1. In a 12-inch skillet, heat oil over medium-high heat. Add chops and cook, turning, until browned on both sides, about 8 minutes. Season with ¼ teaspoon each salt and pepper. Remove chops to a plate. Drain off any fat from skillet.

2. Add 1½ cups tomato sauce, garlic, basil, remaining ¼ teaspoon salt, water, rice, and green pepper to skillet; blend thoroughly. Heat to boiling over high heat, stirring occasionally. Place chops on top of mixture. Reduce heat to medium-low, cover, and simmer 20 minutes.

3. Carefully stir in green beans. Arrange a slice of mozzarella cheese on each chop, top with remaining tomato sauce, and sprinkle Parmesan cheese over all. Cover and simmer 8 to 10 minutes, or until pork chops and beans are tender and cheese is melted.

122   SKILLET SAUSAGE AND RED CABBAGE WITH CORN AND PEPPERS

Prep: 10 minutes   Cook: 20 to 24 minutes   Serves: 4 to 5

This combination of ingredients may surprise you, but the sausage and red cabbage are delicious partners. The dish is not only interesting, but attractive as well.

1 pound fully cooked Polish kielbasa sausage, thinly sliced	1 small green bell pepper, cut into thin strips
1 medium head red cabbage, shredded	2 cups frozen corn kernels, thawed
1 small red bell pepper, cut into thin strips	¼ cup red wine vinegar Dash of cayenne

1. Heat a 10-inch skillet until hot. Add half of sausage and cook over medium heat, stirring occasionally, until lightly browned, 6 to 8 minutes; remove to a plate. Add remaining sausage and cook until brown; remove to same plate. Drain off all but about 1 tablespoon sausage drippings from pan.

2. Add red cabbage and cook over medium heat, stirring often, for 6 to 8 minutes, or until wilted.

3. Add red and green peppers and cook, stirring, until slightly softened, 3 to 4 minutes. Stir in corn, vinegar, and cayenne. Heat to boiling. Reduce heat to medium and cook another 4 or 5 minutes, or until cabbage is tender. Return sausage to skillet, stir in, cover, and heat through.

123   SAUSAGE, PEPPER, AND POTATO MEDLEY
Prep: 10 minutes   Cook: 21 to 26 minutes   Serves: 4 to 5

If you have a craving for potatoes, here's one way to cook them fast. Team them up with sausage slices (use the light varieties for less fat) and red and green pepper strips for an appealing entrée.

1½ **pounds fully cooked Polish kielbasa sausage**
2 **medium onions, quartered and sliced**
5 **medium baking potatoes, peeled and diced**
⅓ **cup water**

½ **teaspoon salt**
1 **red bell pepper, cut into thin 1-inch-long strips**
1 **green bell pepper, cut into thin 1-inch long strips**
¼ **teaspoon pepper**

1. Cut sausage into ½-inch diagonal slices.

2. In a 10- to 12-inch skillet, cook sausage and onions over medium-high heat, stirring often, until onions are golden, 6 to 8 minutes. Drain off any excess fat that accumulates.

3. Stir in potatoes, water, and salt. Heat to boiling. Reduce heat to medium, cover, and cook 10 minutes.

4. Stir in red and green peppers. Cook, covered, over medium heat, 5 to 8 minutes, or until potatoes are tender. Season with pepper.

124 RISOTTO WITH ITALIAN SAUSAGE
Prep: 10 minutes   Cook: 25 minutes   Serves: 6 to 8

Arborio rice, imported from Italy, is available in Italian specialty markets as well as many supermarkets. Short and plump and coated with a starch that creates a creamy smooth sauce, it is essential to a true risotto.

1 pound sweet or hot Italian
  sausage
1 tablespoon olive oil
1 tablespoon butter
1 medium onion, chopped
1 pound Arborio rice
2 cups simmering water
1 (14½-ounce) can beef broth
1 (14½-ounce) can cut-up,
  peeled tomatoes,
  undrained

¼ pound fresh mushrooms,
  sliced
1 (6-ounce) jar sweet fried
  peppers with onions,
  drained
3 tablespoons grated
  Parmesan cheese

1. In a 12-inch skillet, place sausages with enough cold water to cover. Heat to boiling over high heat. Reduce heat to medium, cover, and cook 10 minutes.

2. Drain and discard water from sausages. Place sausages on a cutting board.

3. In same skillet, heat oil and butter over medium-high heat until butter is melted. Add onion and cook until limp, 2 to 3 minutes.

4. Add rice and cook, stirring, 1 minute. Stir in 1 cup water and continue to cook, stirring, until water has almost evaporated, about 2 minutes. Add an additional 1 cup water and cook, stirring, until water is absorbed, about 3 minutes. Add broth and cook, stirring, until broth has been absorbed by rice, 5 to 7 minutes.

5. Add tomatoes with their liquid and cook, stirring, until juice has been absorbed, about 2 minutes. Stir in mushrooms and drained peppers. Reduce heat to low.

6. Slice sausages and add to skillet; mix in. Sprinkle with cheese and serve immediately.

125   SAUSAGE-RICE SKILLET WITH BROCCOLI
Prep: 5 minutes   Cook: 35 minutes   Serves: 4 to 5

When you're tired after a busy day, toss this dish together and relax for half an hour while it cooks. Use any combination of frozen vegetables that suits your palate.

¾ **pound fully cooked Polish kielbasa sausage, sliced into ¼-inch-thick rounds**
3 **scallions, chopped**
1 **cup converted rice**
1 **(14½-ounce) can beef broth**
1 **(16-ounce) package frozen broccoli, corn, and red peppers**

1 **(10-ounce) package frozen cut broccoli spears**
½ **teaspoon garlic powder**
¼ **teaspoon salt**
¼ **teaspoon pepper**

1. In a 10-inch skillet, cook sausage over medium-high heat, stirring occasionally, until browned, 8 to 10 minutes. Drain off any fat.

2. Stir in scallions, rice, broth, frozen vegetables, garlic powder, salt, and pepper. Heat to boiling, stirring occasionally. Reduce heat to medium-low, cover, and simmer 25 minutes, or until liquid is absorbed and rice is tender.

126   SPICY GERMAN BRATWURST
Prep: 30 minutes   Cook: 1¾ hours   Serves: 4 to 6

When only hearty fare to warm the soul will suffice, this is a good choice.

2 **pounds fresh German bratwurst sausages (8 to 10 links)**
1 **(12-ounce) bottle lager beer**
½ **cup chili sauce**
1 **tablespoon Worcestershire sauce**
½ **cup ketchup**
½ **cup cider vinegar**
½ **cup lightly packed brown sugar**

1 **teaspoon paprika**
1 **teaspoon ground nutmeg**
2 **medium onions, cut into ¼-inch slices, rings separated**
3 **russet potatoes, peeled and thinly sliced**
½ **teaspoon salt**
¼ **teaspoon pepper**

1. Prick bratwurst with a fork. In a 12-inch skillet, cook bratwurst in enough water to cover over medium-high heat 15 minutes. Remove bratwurst to a plate and discard water.

2. In same skillet, combine beer, chili sauce, Worcestershire sauce, ketchup, vinegar, brown sugar, paprika, and nutmeg. Heat to boiling; reduce heat to low. Layer onions and potatoes with bratwurst in sauce. Season with salt and pepper. Cover and simmer 1½ hours.

127 SAUSAGE AND VEGETABLE HERO SANDWICH

Prep: 10 minutes   Cook: 50 minutes   Serves: 4 to 5

Hot Italian sausage and vegetables combine for a delicious hot supper sandwich served on split French rolls.

½ pound hot Italian sausage links
½ pound sweet Italian sausage links
½ cup water
2 medium onions, quartered and sliced
2 medium green bell peppers, cut into thin strips

1 medium red bell pepper, cut into thin strips
2 medium zucchini, chopped
2 garlic cloves, minced
1½ teaspoons basil
½ teaspoon oregano
½ cup dry white wine
4 to 5 (7- to 8-inch) French rolls, split and toasted

1. Place sausage links in a 10-inch skillet. Add water and cook, uncovered, over medium-high heat, turning occasionally, until water evaporates, about 10 minutes. Reduce heat to low and continue cooking, turning occasionally, until sausages are lightly browned, about 5 minutes.

2. Remove sausages to a cutting board; cut diagonally into ¼-inch slices. Return to skillet and cook, over medium heat, stirring, 8 to 10 minutes, or until well browned. Remove to a dish.

3. In same skillet, cook onions over medium heat, stirring occasionally, 4 to 5 minutes, or until limp. Add red and green peppers and zucchini and cook, stirring occasionally, until zucchini is tender, about 10 minutes.

4. Add browned sausage, garlic, basil, oregano, and wine. Heat to boiling, reduce heat to low, and simmer 10 minutes. To serve, place a split roll on individual serving plates and spoon some of sausage and vegetable mixture on one or both halves. Serve immediately.

128 SWEET POTATOES, HAM, AND APPLES A L'ORANGE

Prep: 10 minutes   Cook: 15 minutes   Serves: 4

This interesting entrée combines cooked ham (use leftovers if you have some handy) with sweet potatoes, apples, and orange juice for a terrific and simple meal-in-a-skillet. Serve with coleslaw or a green vegetable salad.

2 large sweet potatoes, peeled and thinly sliced (about 4 cups)
2 Granny Smith apples, cored and chopped
1 medium onion, chopped

¾ cup orange juice
½ teaspoon ground cinnamon
2 cups diced cooked ham or turkey ham
⅓ cup chopped pecans

1. In a 10-inch skillet, combine sweet potatoes, apples, and onion. Pour

½ cup orange juice over all. Heat to boiling. Reduce heat to medium, cover, and steam 8 to 10 minutes, until potatoes are almost tender.

2. Remove cover, stir in remaining ¼ cup orange juice, cinnamon, and ham until well mixed. Heat through 5 minutes, or until hot. Serve sprinkled with chopped pecans.

---

129 SPICED LAMB WITH CABBAGE AND BACON

Prep: 25 minutes   Cook: 2¼ hours   Serves: 6 to 8

This lamb creation is fragrant with spices and a hint of orange.

2 pounds boneless lamb, cut into ½-inch cubes	1 pound green cabbage, finely shredded
1 teaspoon salt	1 teaspoon ground cinnamon
¼ teaspoon pepper	½ teaspoon ground allspice
4 thick bacon slices, diced	½ teaspoon ground cloves
¼ cup olive oil	Grated zest of 2 oranges
2 medium onions, chopped	1 cup fresh orange juice
2 garlic cloves, minced	1 cup sour cream
1 tablespoon flour	½ cup chopped walnuts
4 cups beef stock or canned broth	6 toasted bread slices, cut into triangles to make toast points
¼ cup chopped parsley	
2 tablespoons chopped fresh mint, or 1½ teaspoons dried	

1. Season lamb with ¼ teaspoon each salt and pepper.

2. In a 12-inch skillet, cook bacon over medium-high heat, stirring occasionally, until crisp, 3 to 5 minutes. Drain off fat.

3. Add oil to bacon in skillet and heat over medium-high heat until hot. Add lamb and cook, tossing occasionally, until brown on all sides, 6 to 8 minutes.

4. Add onions and garlic and cook, stirring occasionally, until soft, 2 to 3 minutes. Mix in flour well. Cook, stirring, 2 minutes.

5. Whisk in beef broth and remaining ¾ teaspoon salt. Heat to boiling over high heat, stirring occasionally. Cover, reduce heat to low, and simmer 1½ hours.

6. Stir in parsley, mint, cabbage, cinnamon, allspice, cloves, orange zest, and orange juice. Simmer, covered, 20 minutes longer. Stir in sour cream and simmer until heated through but not boiling, about 2 minutes. Fold in walnuts. Serve over toast points.

130   PIZZA RICE SKILLET
Prep: 10 minutes   Cook: 30 minutes   Serves: 4

For a dish that's appealing to children, try this stove-top entrée with a vegetable-rice base and the flavors of pizza atop it all. Vary the toppings, pizza style, to suit individual tastes.

1 tablespoon butter	1 (4-ounce) can mushroom
1½ cups shredded zucchini	stems and pieces, drained
1 large onion, chopped	1 (2.2-ounce) can sliced ripe
2 cups boiling water	olives, drained
1 cup converted rice	1 to 1½ cups shredded
¾ teaspoon Italian seasoning	mozzarella or cheddar
¾ cup pizza sauce or tomato	cheese
sauce	
12 slices salami, or ¾ cup	
cut-up cooked chicken	

1. In a 10-inch skillet, melt butter over medium-high heat. Add zucchini and onion and cook, stirring, until soft, about 5 minutes.

2. Stir in boiling water, rice, and Italian seasoning. Heat to boiling, reduce heat to low, cover, and simmer about 20 minutes, until rice is almost tender.

3. Spread pizza sauce evenly over rice, then arrange salami slices on top. Sprinkle with mushrooms, olives, and cheese. Cover skillet and cook over medium heat about 5 minutes, until cheese is melted.

131   EMERGENCY RICE AND FRANK SKILLET SUPPER
Prep: 5 minutes   Cook: 15 minutes   Serves: 4 to 5

When time is short and you need to get something on the table fast, this is one possibility—and it's appealing to children.

1 (28-ounce) can crushed	2 cups instant rice
tomatoes with added	2 tablespoons grated
puree	Parmesan cheese
½ green bell pepper, chopped	(optional)
¾ pound beef franks, sliced	¾ cup shredded mozzarella
½ inch thick	cheese
1½ teaspoons basil	

1. In a large skillet, combine tomatoes, green pepper, franks, and basil. Heat to boiling, stirring occasionally. Stir in rice. Cover pan and remove from heat.

2. Let stand 5 to 10 minutes, until liquid is absorbed and rice is tender. Stir with fork to fluff.

3. Stir in Parmesan cheese. Sprinkle mozzarella cheese over top, cover, and cook over low heat 5 minutes, or until cheese melts.

132 SHRIMP WITH GREEN BEANS, TOMATOES, AND FETA CHEESE

Prep: 10 minutes   Cook: 15 minutes   Serves: 4

2 tablespoons olive oil
1 pound medium shrimp, shelled and deveined
3 large garlic cloves, crushed through a press
1½ pounds fresh green beans, trimmed and cut into 1-inch lengths

1 (28-ounce) can peeled tomatoes, well drained and cut up
2 tablespoons dry white wine
2 tablespoons fresh lemon juice
1 cup crumbled feta cheese (about 8 ounces)

1. In a 10- or 12-inch skillet, heat 1 tablespoon oil over high heat. Add shrimp and garlic and cook, tossing frequently, until shrimp are pink and loosely curled, 2 to 3 minutes. Remove shrimp to a plate.

2. Add remaining 1 tablespoon oil to skillet and, when melted, add green beans, tomatoes, and wine. Heat to boiling, stirring once or twice. Reduce heat to medium, cover, and cook about 10 minutes, until beans are crisp-tender.

3. Return shrimp to skillet. Stir in lemon juice and feta. Cook until heated through, about 1 minute. Serve over hot cooked rice or pasta.

133 WILD RICE WITH SHRIMP AND CILANTRO

Prep: 20 minutes   Cook: 25 minutes   Serves: 4

1 pound frozen cooked, peeled, deveined medium shrimp
2 tablespoons olive oil
1 medium onion, chopped
1 medium red bell pepper, chopped
1 medium green bell pepper, chopped
3 garlic cloves, mashed
2 cups hot water

1 (9-ounce) package brown and white Texmati rice blend with wild rice
Juice of 2 limes
½ teaspoon salt
¼ teaspoon pepper
1 large head fresh romaine lettuce, shredded
2 medium tomatoes, quartered
½ cup chopped fresh cilantro

1. Rinse frozen shrimp in a colander with cold water; set aside to drain.

2. In a 12-inch skillet or large flameproof casserole, heat oil until hot. Add onion and red and green peppers and cook, stirring occasionally, until limp, about 5 minutes. Stir in garlic, hot water, and rice; mix well. Heat to boiling; stir. Reduce heat to medium-low, cover, and cook 15 minutes.

3. Stir in lime juice, shrimp, salt, and pepper. Cover and cook 5 to 7 minutes longer. Serve, mounding slightly, on lettuce-lined plates with tomatoes. Sprinkle with cilantro.

134 SAUCY SHRIMP WITH ARTICHOKES
Prep: 15 minutes   Cook: 20 minutes   Serves: 6

An easy shrimp and artichoke dish.

4 tablespoons butter
1 (9-ounce) package frozen
   artichokes, thawed
1½ pounds medium shrimp,
   shelled and deveined
2¾ cups water
⅓ cup dry white wine
1 teaspoon powdered chicken
   stock base

2 (4.5-ounce) packages rice
   and sauce, chicken flavor
½ cup chopped red bell pepper
3 scallions, chopped
1 (10-ounce) package frozen
   French-style green beans,
   thawed

1. In a 12-inch skillet, melt butter over medium heat. Add artichokes and cook, stirring occasionally, 2 minutes.

2. Add shrimp, increase heat to high, and cook, stirring, 2 to 3 minutes, or until shrimp are pink and loosely curled.

3. Add water, wine, chicken stock base, and rice mixes. Heat to boiling over high heat; boil 1 minute. Reduce heat to low and simmer, uncovered, 5 minutes.

4. Stir in red peppers, scallions, and green beans. Cook over medium-low heat 5 to 8 minutes longer, or until rice is tender and beans are cooked through. Serve immediately.

135 CREAMY MUSTARD SHRIMP WITH VEGETABLES
Prep: 10 minutes   Cook: 20 minutes   Serves: 4

With its mustard and white wine sauce and a mélange of vegetables, this dish is special enough for a company meal.

4 tablespoons butter
8 carrots, peeled and cut into
   thin strips
2 leeks, washed well and cut
   into thin strips
3 zucchini, cut into thin strips
½ pound fresh mushrooms,
   sliced
2 tablespoons vegetable oil
1 pound peeled and deveined
   large shrimp

½ teaspoon salt
¼ teaspoon pepper
½ cup dry white wine
½ cup heavy cream
1½ tablespoons Dijon mustard
1 tablespoon Pommery or
   other grainy mustard
2 tablespoons snipped chives
   or chopped fresh
   watercress (optional)

1. In a 12-inch skillet, melt 2 tablespoons butter over medium-high heat. Add carrots, leeks, zucchini, and mushrooms. Cook, stirring, 5 minutes. Reduce heat to low, cover, and cook until carrots are crisp-tender, about 5 minutes longer. Remove vegetables to a plate and cover with foil to keep warm.

2. Add remaining 2 tablespoons butter and oil to same skillet and heat until hot over medium-high heat. Add shrimp and season with salt and pepper. Cook, stirring, 2 to 3 minutes, until shrimp turn pink and are loosely curled. Remove to a plate.

3. Add wine and cream to skillet and boil over medium-high heat, stirring occasionally, about 5 minutes to reduce and thicken sauce slightly.

4. Stir in Dijon and Pommery mustards, shrimp, and vegetable mixture. Heat through, about 2 minutes. Garnish with snipped chives.

136   CURRIED SHRIMP, RICE, AND VEGETABLES
Prep: 10 minutes   Cook: 40 to 45 minutes   Serves: 4

This curried shrimp dish is special enough to serve for casual company fare. Sprinkle with shredded coconut and cashews for a festive touch.

1 **tablespoon butter**
1 **leek (white and tender green), washed well and chopped**
1 **cup converted rice**
1 **garlic clove, minced**
1 **to 2 tablespoons Madras curry powder**
1½ **cups hot water**
1 **cup heavy cream**
1 **(16-ounce) package frozen broccoli, cauliflower, and red peppers, partially thawed**

Juice of 1 lime
½ **teaspoon salt**
¼ **teaspoon pepper**
¾ **pound peeled and deveined medium shrimp (thawed and well drained, if frozen)**
⅓ **cup shredded coconut**
⅓ **cup cashews**

1. In a 10-inch skillet, melt butter over medium heat. Add leek and cook, stirring 1 to 2 minutes, until soft. Stir in rice, garlic, and curry powder. Cook, stirring, 3 minutes.

2. Stir in water and cream. Heat to boiling over high heat, stirring occasionally. Reduce heat to low, cover, and simmer 15 minutes.

3. Remove cover and stir in vegetables, breaking them up. Increase heat to medium. Cover and cook 15 to 20 minutes, or until rice is tender.

4. Stir in lime juice, salt, pepper, and shrimp. Cover and cook 5 to 10 minutes longer, or until shrimp are pink and loosely curled and vegetables are hot. Serve topped with coconut and cashews.

137   SPANISH SHRIMP AND RICE
Prep: 20 minutes   Cook: 30 minutes   Serves: 6

Here's a shrimp variation on the Spanish rice theme, but this version has a slightly soupy consistency.

3 tablespoons vegetable oil
2 cups long-grain white rice
1 medium onion, chopped
2 celery ribs, chopped
1 garlic clove, minced
½ cup chopped green bell
   pepper
1 pound medium shrimp,
   shelled and deveined
1 teaspoon ground cumin

1 teaspoon salt
½ teaspoon pepper
2 (10-ounce) cans diced
   tomatoes and green
   chiles, undrained
1 (4-ounce) can diced green
   chiles
2½ cups chicken broth
1 cup frozen peas, thawed

1. In a 12-inch skillet, heat oil until hot over medium-high heat. Add rice and cook, stirring occasionally, until light beige colored, 3 to 4 minutes.

2. Stir in onion, celery, garlic, and green pepper. Cook until onion is just soft, 2 to 3 minutes.

3. Add shrimp, cumin, salt, and pepper. Cook, stirring constantly, until shrimp are pink, 2 to 3 minutes.

4. Stir in tomatoes with their liquid, green chiles, and broth. Heat to boiling over high heat. Reduce heat to low, stir, cover, and simmer 10 minutes.

5. Sprinkle peas over top. Cover and cook for 10 minutes, or until rice is tender. Dish should have some liquid remaining for a slightly soupy consistency. Stir peas into rice.

138   WARM PEAR AND SCALLOP SALAD
Prep: 20 minutes   Cook: 10 minutes   Serves: 4

2 carrots, peeled and cut into
   thin strips
1 zucchini, cut into thin strips
1 potato, peeled and cut into
   thin strips
1 pound sea scallops
3 fresh firm ripe pears, cored
   and cut into 1-inch
   chunks

½ cup chopped pecans
½ cup bottled ranch-style salad
   dressing
6 to 7 cups mixed salad greens
1 large tomato, cut into 8 slices

1. In a 10- or 12-inch skillet, combine carrot, zucchini, and potato strips with enough cold water to cover. Heat to boiling, cover, and cook for 4 to 5 minutes, until just tender. Add scallops and cook until just opaque throughout, about 2 minutes. Drain and discard liquid.

2. Remove pan from heat. Add pears, pecans, and dressing and toss to combine. Serve over salad greens on individual serving plates with 2 tomato slices on each salad.

---

139 SPANISH SCALLOPS AND RICE
Prep: 10 minutes   Cook: 30 to 35 minutes   Serves: 4 to 5

Combine frozen scallops with a package of rice mix for an interesting and easy meal-in-a-dish.

2 tablespoons olive oil
2 tablespoons butter
1 onion, chopped
1 medium red bell pepper, chopped
1 medium yellow bell pepper, chopped
1 (5.3-ounce) package rice and pasta mix with bell peppers, olives, and Mexican seasonings

1 (14½-ounce) can chicken broth
2 teaspoons basil
1 cup heavy cream
1 pound sea scallops
Juice of 2 limes
2 to 3 plum tomatoes, chopped
3 tablespoons chopped fresh cilantro or parsley

1. In a 12-inch skillet, heat oil and butter together over medium-high heat until butter is melted. Add onion and red and yellow peppers and cook, stirring, 3 minutes. Stir in rice and pasta and seasonings from mix, broth, and basil. Cover and reduce heat to medium-low. Cook 20 to 25 minutes, until most of liquid is absorbed.

2. Stir in cream. Cook over medium-high heat, stirring occasionally to avoid scorching, 5 minutes. Add scallops and cook until just opaque throughout, 3 to 5 minutes.

3. Remove from heat and stir in lime juice. Sprinkle top with tomatoes. Garnish with a sprinkling of cilantro.

140   FILLET OF SOLE WITH PORT
Prep: 20 minutes   Cook: 30 minutes   Serves: 4 to 5

White port and cream lend special flavor and flair to this dish, which would make appealing company fare.

2 tablespoons olive oil	¼ teaspoon pepper
¼ pound fresh mushrooms, sliced	1 (10-ounce) package frozen mixed vegetables
4 to 5 scallions, chopped	1 pound fresh sole fillets
1½ cups quick-cooking brown rice	½ cup heavy cream
1 cup water	2 medium tomatoes, chopped
½ cup white port	Grated zest of 1 lemon
½ teaspoon salt	¼ cup chopped parsley

1. In a 12-inch skillet, heat oil over high heat until hot. Add mushrooms and scallions and cook, stirring, 2 minutes.

2. Stir in brown rice, water, port, salt, and pepper. Heat to boiling, reduce heat to low, cover, and simmer 14 minutes.

3. Stir in frozen vegetables. Lay sole on top of mixture. Pour cream over fish. Sprinkle tomatoes, lemon zest, and parsley over fish. Cover and cook over medium heat 10 to 15 minutes, or until fish flakes easily.

141   STEAMED SOLE WITH TOMATO, FENNEL, AND ORZO
Prep: 10 minutes   Cook: 20 minutes   Serves: 4

The marriage of orzo (tiny rice-shaped pasta) and sole with tomato, fennel, and spinach makes this quick dish a winner

1 medium bulb fresh fennel	1½ cups water
1 tablespoon olive oil	2 tablespoons fresh lemon juice
4 scallions, chopped	1 cup orzo (rice-shaped pasta)
2 cups packed chopped fresh spinach	½ teaspoon salt
1 cup chopped fresh or drained canned tomatoes	¼ teaspoon pepper
1 garlic clove, minced	1 pound fresh sole fillets

1. Quarter fennel bulb lengthwise, then cut crosswise into thin slices. Chop feathery green tops and set aside.

2. In a 10-inch skillet, heat oil over high heat until hot. Add scallions and cook, stirring, 2 minutes, until limp. Add sliced fennel, spinach, ¾ cup tomatoes, and garlic. Cook, stirring occasionally, 3 to 4 minutes, until spinach is limp.

3. Stir in water, 1 tablespoon lemon juice, orzo, salt, and pepper. Heat to boiling, stirring occasionally. Place sole in single layer on top of orzo mixture. Sprinkle with remaining 1 tablespoon lemon juice, chopped fennel tops, and remaining ¼ cup tomatoes.

4. Reduce heat to medium-low, cover, and simmer 10 minutes, or until fish is cooked through and orzo is tender.

142 BRAISED HALIBUT WITH VEGETABLES AND RICE

Prep: 10 minutes   Cook: 20 to 25 minutes   Serves: 4 to 5

This is an easy way to cook fish on top of the stove, and it tastes wonderful to boot.

2 tablespoons olive oil
1 leek (white and tender green), washed well and chopped
1 (14½-ounce) can cut-up, peeled tomatoes, undrained
¾ teaspoon fennel seeds
1 (16-ounce) package frozen mixed vegetables

¼ cup orange juice
½ cup quick-cooking long-grain white rice
1 pound halibut steaks, cut ¾- to 1-inch thick
½ teaspoon salt
¼ teaspoon lemon pepper
¼ cup chopped parsley
Lemon wedges

1. In a 10- or 12-inch skillet, heat oil over medium-high heat. Add leeks and cook, stirring, 2 to 3 minutes, until softened but not browned.

2. Stir in tomatoes with their liquid, fennel seeds, mixed vegetables, orange juice, and rice. Heat to boiling, stirring often.

3. Arrange halibut steaks in a single layer on top of vegetable mixture. Season with salt and lemon pepper. Reduce heat to low.

4. Cover and simmer 15 to 17 minutes, turning halibut once, until cooked through. Sprinkle with parsley and serve with lemon wedges.

143   RED SNAPPER AND RICE DINNER
Prep: 10 minutes   Cook: 20 to 25 minutes   Serves: 4 to 5

This is a great way to whip up a fish dinner in a single dish. Vary the kind of fish fillets according to the best-in-season buys your fishmonger is offering.

1 (6.25-ounce) package quick-cooking long-grain and wild rice mix
1¾ cups water
¼ cup dry white wine
1 (16-ounce) package frozen cut broccoli spears

2 carrots, peeled and shredded
Juice and grated zest of 1 lemon
1 pound red snapper fillets
¼ cup chopped parsley

1. In a 10- or 12-inch skillet, combine contents of rice and seasoning packets from rice mix, water, wine, broccoli, carrots, and half the lemon zest. Heat to boiling over high heat, stirring often; boil 1 minute. Spread evenly in skillet.

2. Place snapper in a single layer on top of rice. Sprinkle with remaining lemon zest and half the lemon juice.

3. Reduce heat to medium-low. Cover and simmer 14 to 15 minutes, or until snapper flakes easily and rice is tender. Sprinkle with remaining lemon juice and parsley.

144   QUICK TUNA AND POTATO SKILLET DINNER
Prep: 5 minutes   Cook: 20 to 25 minutes   Serves: 4

This is one of those nothing fancy jiffy skillet dinners, terrific to rely on when you don't feel like cooking. Even the kids will be happy with this choice.

1 (24-ounce) package frozen O'Brien potatoes with onions and peppers
1 cup milk
¼ teaspoon garlic salt

¼ teaspoon pepper
1 cup frozen peas and carrots
1 (6½- or 7-ounce) can tuna packed in water, drained
1½ cups grated cheddar cheese

1. In a 10-inch skillet, combine frozen potatoes and milk. Heat to boiling, stirring often to break up potatoes.

2. Cover, reduce heat to low, and simmer 10 to 15 minutes, until potatoes are thawed and tender.

3. Remove cover and stir in garlic salt, pepper, peas and carrots, and tuna. Cook until peas and carrots are tender and tuna is hot, 2 to 3 minutes. Stir in 1 cup cheese, mixing well. Sprinkle remaining ½ cup cheese over top. Cover and cook over low heat until cheese is melted, 2 to 3 minutes.

145   NOODLES CHICKEN DIVAN
Prep: 10 minutes   Cook: 35 minutes   Serves: 6

The flavors of chicken divan are assembled in this stove-top dish that cooks effortlessly while you go about other chores.

1 tablespoon butter	1 cup light cream or half-and-half
1 medium red bell pepper, chopped	3 cups medium noodles (6 ounces)
3 scallions, chopped	1½ cups chopped cooked chicken
4 cups chopped fresh broccoli (1 bunch)	
1 (14½-ounce) can chicken broth	

1. In a large skillet, melt butter over medium heat. Add red pepper, scallions, and broccoli. Cook, stirring occasionally, 5 minutes.

2. Stir in chicken broth, cream, noodles, and chicken. Heat to boiling. Reduce heat to low, cover, and simmer over low heat 25 to 30 minutes, or until noodles are tender.

146   EASY SKILLET LASAGNE
Prep: 10 minutes   Cook: 30 minutes   Serves: 4 to 5

When you desire the flavor of lasagne but have little time, try this quick stove-top version.

1 pound lean ground beef	8 ounces medium egg noodles
1 medium onion, chopped	1 cup ricotta cheese
1 (15-ounce) can herb-flavored tomato sauce	3 tablespoons grated Parmesan cheese
2 cups water	1 egg
2 garlic cloves, minced	2 tablespoons chopped parsley
2 teaspoons basil	¼ teaspoon pepper
½ teaspoon oregano	

1. In a 10-inch skillet, cook beef and onion over medium-high heat, stirring often, until meat is browned, about 5 minutes. Drain off fat.

2. Stir in tomato sauce, water, garlic, basil, oregano, and noodles. Heat to boiling, stirring. Reduce heat to low, cover, and simmer 10 minutes

3. Meanwhile, mix together cheeses, egg, parsley, and pepper. Spoon cheese topping in 5 mounds around edge of skillet and one in center. Cover and simmer 15 minutes longer.

147 SPEEDY STOVE-TOP SPAGHETTI

Prep: 10 minutes   Cook: 32 to 35 minutes   Serves: 6

You won't believe how quickly this spaghetti-in-a-dish is completed.

1 pound sweet Italian sausage, removed from casing and crumbled
1 onion, chopped, or 2 tablespoons instant minced onion
1 garlic clove, crushed
1½ cups broken 1-inch lengths thin spaghetti
1 tablespoon chopped parsley

2 teaspoons basil
1 (28-ounce) can cut-up, peeled tomatoes, undrained
1 (15-ounce) can tomato sauce
3 tablespoons dry red or white wine
3 tablespoons grated Parmesan cheese

1. In a 10- or 12-inch skillet, cook sausage and onion over medium heat, stirring often, until sausage is browned and cooked through, 5 to 7 minutes. Drain off any excess fat.

2. Stir in garlic and broken spaghetti and cook, stirring, 5 minutes.

3. Stir in all remaining ingredients except Parmesan cheese until well mixed. Heat to boiling. Reduce heat to low, cover, and simmer about 20 minutes, until spaghetti is tender. Sprinkle with Parmesan cheese. Cover and cook 2 to 3 minutes longer to melt cheese.

148 TOMATO AND BROCCOLI PASTA

Prep: 10 minutes   Cook: 20 minutes   Serves: 3

1½ tablespoons olive oil
1 small onion, chopped
2 garlic cloves, minced
2 tablespoons minced parsley
½ cup chopped fresh basil, or 1 tablespoon dried
1 teaspoon salt
1 teaspoon sugar
¼ to ½ teaspoon crushed hot red pepper flakes

3 tablespoons tomato paste
1 (28-ounce) can crushed tomatoes with added puree
½ cup quartered ripe olives
2 cups broccoli florets
8 ounces corkscrew noodles, cooked and drained
¼ cup grated Parmesan cheese

1. In a 10-inch skillet, heat oil over moderate heat until hot. Add onion and garlic and cook, stirring occasionally, until onion is soft, about 3 minutes.

2. Stir in parsley, basil, salt, sugar, hot pepper, tomato paste, tomatoes with puree, and olives. Heat to boiling, reduce heat to low, and simmer 10 minutes. Mix in broccoli, cover, and simmer until broccoli is tender, about 5 minutes.

3. Serve sauce over hot cooked noodles. Top with Parmesan cheese.

149 SIMPLE SPAGHETTI MAC
Prep: 5 minutes   Cook: 35 to 42 minutes   Serves: 6

Produce this dinner in a skillet effortlessly. While you're waiting for it to cook, whip up a green salad with a few assorted vegetables to accompany it.

1 pound hot or sweet Italian
    sausage or lean ground
    beef, or a combination of
    the two
1 medium onion, chopped
1 (27½-ounce) can spaghetti
    sauce with mushrooms

2 teaspoons basil
¾ cup water
¾ cup dry white wine
1½ cups elbow macaroni
2 cups chopped fresh spinach
    or Swiss chard (optional)

1. Remove sausage from casings and crumble into a 10- or 12-inch skillet along with onion. Cook over medium heat, stirring often, until sausage is browned and cooked through, 5 to 7 minutes. Drain off excess fat.

2. Stir in spaghetti sauce, basil, water, and wine; blend well. Mix in macaroni and spinach. Heat to boiling. Reduce heat to low, cover, and cook 30 to 35 minutes, or until macaroni is tender.

150 BOLOGNESE MEAT SAUCE WITH SPAGHETTI
Prep: 10 minutes   Cook: 35 minutes   Serves: 4 to 5

This is a variation on the classic meat sauce, which is native to northern Italy. Instead of pancetta, this version uses bacon. A touch of cream lightens the color of the traditional red sauce.

6 bacon slices, diced
1 pound lean ground beef
1 medium onion, chopped
1 celery rib, chopped
2 carrots, peeled and chopped
1 (28-ounce) can crushed
    tomatoes with added
    puree
2 garlic cloves, minced

1 teaspoon salt
¼ teaspoon pepper
½ cup dry white wine
⅓ cup heavy cream
¾ pound spaghetti, cooked
    until tender
    Grated Parmesan cheese
    (optional)

1. In a 10-inch skillet, fry bacon and beef over medium-high heat until bacon is crisp and beef is brown, about 5 minutes. Drain off excess fat. Add onion, celery, and carrots and cook, stirring often, until onion is tender, about 5 minutes longer.

2. Stir in tomatoes, garlic, salt, and pepper. Heat to boiling, reduce heat to medium-low, cover, and simmer 15 minutes.

3. Mix in wine and cream until well blended. Simmer, uncovered, 10 minutes longer. Serve over hot spaghetti and sprinkle with Parmesan cheese.

151 SKILLET PASTA WITH SHRIMP, SCALLOPS, AND VEGETABLES

Prep: 10 minutes   Cook: 10 minutes   Serves: 3 to 4

This dish is a good one for those watching their calories.

1 tablespoon vegetable oil
3 small zucchini, cut into thin strips
1 medium red bell pepper, slivered
1 medium yellow bell pepper, slivered
1 medium green bell pepper, slivered
1 small red onion, thinly sliced

2 tablespoons finely chopped parsley
1 (8-ounce) bottle clam juice
⅓ cup heavy cream (optional)
½ pound bay scallops
6 ounces bay shrimp
¼ teaspoon salt
Dash of cayenne
1 (9-ounce) package fresh angel hair pasta, cooked and drained

1. In a 10- or 12-inch skillet, heat oil over medium heat. Add zucchini, bell peppers, and red onion. Stir to coat with oil. Cover and cook, stirring occasionally, until vegetables are crisp-tender, 3 to 5 minutes.

2. Add parsley, clam juice, cream, and scallops. Cook, stirring occasionally, until scallops are just opaque throughout, about 3 minutes. Add shrimp and heat through, 1 minute. Season with salt and cayenne.

3. Spoon sauce over hot cooked pasta.

152 GARDEN FRITTATA

Prep: 10 minutes   Cook: 15 to 20 minutes   Serves: 3 to 4

Serve this for brunch or a quick supper.

2 tablespoons olive or vegetable oil
1 cup chopped peeled potatoes (about 2 small)
1 cup shredded zucchini
1 medium green bell pepper, cut into thin strips about 1½ inches long
1 medium red bell pepper, cut into thin strips about 1½ inches long

4 scallions, chopped
1 cup sliced fresh mushrooms
6 eggs
2 tablespoons milk
2 tablespoons grated Parmesan cheese
1 teaspoon basil
½ teaspoon salt
¼ teaspoon pepper

1. In a 10-inch skillet, heat oil over medium heat until hot. Add potatoes, zucchini, green and red pepper, scallions, and mushrooms. Cook over medium heat, stirring often, until vegetables are soft, 5 to 8 minutes. Spread vegetables in an even layer with back of spoon or fork.

2. In a medium bowl, beat together eggs, milk, cheese, basil, salt, and pepper until well mixed. Pour eggs over vegetable mixture in skillet. Prick egg mixture in a few places with a fork and gently lift edges to allow uncooked egg to flow underneath. Do not stir. Cover and cook over low heat 10 to 12 minutes, or until eggs are set.

3. Invert frittata onto serving platter and cut into wedges. Or serve cut into wedges from pan.

153 CHICKEN, SAUSAGE, AND SWEET PEPPERS PASTA
Prep: 10 minutes   Cook: 25 to 30 minutes   Serves: 5 to 6

Simple and fresh tasting, this meal-in-a-skillet is a breeze to whip together.

- 12 ounces penne or other tubular pasta
- 4 skinless, boneless chicken breast halves, cut into thin strips
- ¾ pound sweet or hot Italian sausage, removed from casing
- 1 medium red bell pepper, cut into thin strips
- 1 medium green bell pepper, cut into thin strips
- 1 medium onion, quartered and sliced
- 1 medium bulb fresh fennel, trimmed and chopped (chop and reserve feathery green fronds for garnish)
- 2 large tomatoes, chopped
- 1 garlic clove, minced
- 3 tablespoons chopped fresh basil
- 3 tablespoons dry white wine
- ½ teaspoon salt
- ¼ teaspoon pepper

1. In a deep 10-inch skillet or flameproof casserole, cook pasta in boiling salted water until almost tender, about 10 minutes. Drain well. Set pasta aside on a serving platter and cover with foil to keep warm.

2. In same skillet, cook chicken and sausages over medium heat, stirring often, until sausage is browned and cooked through, 10 to 12 minutes. Drain off any fat.

3. Add red and green peppers, onion, and fennel to skillet. Increase heat to medium-high and cook until peppers are crisp-tender, 3 to 5 minutes. Stir in tomatoes, garlic, basil, wine, salt, and pepper. Reduce heat to medium and cook 2 to 3 minutes, or until hot. Serve sauce over penne and garnish with reserved fennel fronds.

154   CHEESE QUESADILLA
Prep: 5 minutes   Cook: 5 to 10 minutes   Serves: 2 to 4

8 teaspoons vegetable oil
4 (7½- or 8-inch) flour tortillas
1 cup shredded Monterey Jack
   cheese
½ cup canned diced green
   chiles

1 cup canned or homemade
   chili con carne, heated
   Salsa, guacamole, and sour
   cream (optional)

1. Make each quesadilla as follows: Pour 2 teaspoons oil in a large skillet and heat until hot. Lay a tortilla atop oil, swirl around, and turn over.

2. Place ¼ cup grated cheese, 2 tablespoons green chiles, and ¼ cup chili con carne on one half of tortilla. Cook over medium-low heat, covered, until tortilla is golden brown on underside. Fold tortilla in half and remove from pan. Repeat procedure with remaining tortillas.

3. To serve, cut each quesadilla into 4 wedges. Serve with salsa, guacamole, and sour cream on the side.

155   VEGETABLE TOSTADA
Prep: 10 minutes   Cook: 20 minutes   Serves: 4 to 5

Contrast the heat of vegetables with cold crisp lettuce for a simple and quick entrée. Omit the beef, if you'd prefer a meatless version. Or prepare the dish with leftover cooked meats.

½ pound lean ground beef
4 cups sliced zucchini
4 cups sliced yellow summer
   squash and/or pattypan
1 (12-ounce) jar mild green
   chile salsa

½ to ¾ head iceberg lettuce,
   shredded
1 cup shredded Monterey Jack
   or cheddar cheese
½ cup sour cream
½ cup tortilla chips

1. In a 10-inch skillet, cook beef over medium-high heat, stirring to break up lumps, until browned, about 7 minutes. Drain off any fat.

2. Add squash. Cook, stirring, 3 minutes. Stir in 1 cup salsa and heat to boiling. Reduce heat to low, cover, and simmer until squash is crisp-tender, 6 to 8 minutes.

3. Spoon hot mixture over shredded lettuce on individual plates. Top with a sprinkling of cheese, some of remaining salsa, sour cream, and tortilla chips. Serve immediately.

Chapter 4

Stove to Oven: Ovenproof Skillets and Flameproof Casseroles

This chapter deals with recipes that go from stove top to oven. These dishes utilize a single ovenproof skillet (with a handle that won't burn) or a flameproof gratin dish or casserole—that is, a dish that can be used not only in the oven, but over direct heat. The inexpensive utensil that I found worked splendidly during testing was a 9-inch in diameter round Pyroceram (Visions) chicken fryer, or skillet, that was 3 inches deep. A 12x3-inch stainless steel chicken fryer with an ovenproof handle also came in handy for cooking larger quantities of food. Although chicken fryers are extremely versatile with sides higher than regular skillets (to help prevent spattering), these utensils aren't as popular as they once were. However, I had no trouble locating them. Other utensils with the same volume would work equally well with the recipes that follow.

What's innovative about these recipes is that you truly use only a single dish. There's no browning in one pan and then transferring the mixture to another casserole. Spinach Noodle Bake is an adaptation of an old family favorite that's been around for years. Mushroom-Barley Vegetable Bake is a meatless choice with pizazz. Other recipes on the theme include Custard-Baked Beef and Black-Eyed Peas, Chinese Pork Casserole, Tex-Mex Turkey Stuffing Bake, Chicken Pot Pie Deluxe, and many more.

156   EASY BEEFY BEAN BAKE
Prep: 10 minutes   Cook: 45 to 55 minutes   Serves: 6

¼ pound bacon, diced
1 pound lean ground beef
1 medium onion, chopped
⅔ cup hickory-flavored
   barbecue sauce
2 tablespoons prepared
   yellow mustard
2 teaspoons Worcestershire
   sauce

1 (32-ounce) can baked beans,
   fat rind removed,
   undrained
1 (29-ounce) can pinto beans,
   rinsed and drained
3 cups chopped fresh mustard
   greens, Swiss chard, or
   spinach

1. Preheat oven to 350°. In a 2½-quart ovenproof skillet or flameproof casserole, cook bacon, beef, and onion over medium-high heat, stirring occasionally, until bacon is crisp and beef is browned, 5 to 7 minutes. Drain off excess fat.

2. Stir in barbecue sauce, mustard, and Worcestershire sauce until well blended. Add baked beans, pinto beans, and mustard greens. Stir gently to mix.

3. Bake, uncovered, 35 to 45 minutes, or until very hot in center and bubbly.

157   EASY HAMBURGER CASSEROLE
Prep: 10 minutes   Cook: 35 minutes   Serves: 6

This easy casserole is a winner. Keep it in mind for your next potluck offering, too.

1 pound lean ground beef
1 (10-ounce) package frozen
   peas, thawed
2 cups diagonally sliced celery
1 (10¾-ounce) can condensed
   cream of mushroom soup
3 tablespoons milk or dry
   sherry

3 scallions, chopped
3 tablespoons chopped
   pimiento
½ teaspoon salt
½ teaspoon pepper
1 cup crushed potato chips

1. Preheat oven to 375°. In a deep 9-inch ovenproof skillet or a 1½-quart flameproof casserole, cook beef on top of stove over medium-high heat, stirring often, until brown and crumbly, about 5 minutes. Drain off excess fat. Spread meat evenly in skillet. Arrange peas evenly over beef, then sprinkle celery over all.

2. In a medium bowl, mix together undiluted soup, milk, scallions, pimiento, salt, and pepper; pour evenly over celery. Sprinkle potato chips over top.

3. Bake 30 minutes, or until hot and bubbly.

158 UPSIDE-DOWN SKILLET PIZZA
Prep: 10 minutes   Cook: 30 minutes   Serves: 4

Here's a way to get all the flavors of a pizza in one dish, but upside down.

1 **pound lean ground beef**
4 **scallions, chopped**
1 **(14-ounce) jar pizza sauce**
1 **(4½-ounce) jar sliced
   mushrooms, rinsed and
   drained**

½ **green bell pepper, chopped**
1 **cup shredded mozzarella
   cheese (4 ounces)**
½ **cup flour**
½ **cup milk**
1 **egg**

1. Preheat oven to 425°. In a deep 9-inch or a 10-inch ovenproof skillet, cook crumbled beef and scallions over medium-high heat, stirring to break up meat, until beef is browned, 5 to 7 minutes. Drain off any excess fat. Stir in pizza sauce, mushrooms, and green pepper. Simmer 3 minutes.

2. Sprinkle ½ cup cheese over meat mixture. In a bowl, whisk together flour, milk, and egg until well blended. Stir in remaining ½ cup cheese. Spread batter evenly over meat mixture and cheese.

3. Bake 20 minutes, or until light golden. Cut into wedges to serve.

159 HAMBURGER-TAMALE CASSEROLE
Prep: 15 minutes   Cook: 45 minutes   Serves: 4 to 5

This is a great choice to tote to a potluck supper—and it's easy on the cook.

1 **pound lean ground beef**
1 **medium onion, chopped**
½ **teaspoon garlic powder**
1 **(8-ounce) can tomato sauce**
1 **(7-ounce) can green chile
   salsa**
1 **(12-ounce) can corn kernels
   with red and green sweet
   peppers, drained**

1 **(2.2-ounce) can sliced ripe
   olives, drained**
4 **(3-ounce) packages prepared
   refrigerated beef tamales**
1 **cup grated cheddar cheese**
3 **tablespoons chopped fresh
   cilantro or parsley**

1. Preheat oven to 350°. In a 10-inch ovenproof skillet or flameproof casserole, cook beef and onion over medium-high heat, stirring occasionally, until beef is browned, 5 to 7 minutes. Drain off fat.

2. Add garlic powder, tomato sauce, salsa, corn and peppers, and olives. Stir to mix well. Cut tamales crosswise into quarters and gently submerge in beef mixture, spacing them evenly.

3. Cover and bake 30 minutes. Uncover; sprinkle cheese over top and bake 10 minutes longer. Garnish with cilantro before serving.

160   BEEF AND POTATO CASSEROLE
Prep: 5 minutes   Cook: 43 to 45 minutes   Serves: 6

This meal-in-a-dish requires minimal effort to get into the oven.

1 **pound lean ground beef**
4 **scallions, chopped**
1 **(16-ounce) package frozen mixed vegetables, thawed and drained**
1 **(10¾-ounce) can condensed cream of celery soup**
1 **(10¾-ounce) can condensed cream of mushroom soup**
1 **(16-ounce) package Tater Tots (seasoned shredded potatoes)**

1. Preheat oven to 375°. In a 10-inch ovenproof skillet or flameproof casserole, cook beef over medium-high heat, stirring often, until brown and crumbly, 5 to 7 minutes. Drain off excess fat. Add scallions and cook 3 minutes longer.

2. Stir in vegetables and undiluted soups; mix well. Top with Tater Tots, arranging evenly over beef mixture.

3. Bake about 35 minutes, or until bubbly and potatoes are crisp and browned.

161   BAKED SKILLET TAMALE PIE
Prep: 10 minutes   Cook: 35 minutes   Serves: 4 to 5

This tamale pie variation sports a cornbread topping. Start the dish stovetop, then add the cornbread batter and pop it in the oven.

1 **pound lean ground beef**
1 **onion, chopped**
1 **green bell pepper, chopped**
1 **(14½-ounce) can cut-up, peeled tomatoes, undrained**
1 **(8-ounce) can tomato sauce**
1 **(12-ounce) can corn kernels, drained**
1 **(2.2-ounce) can sliced ripe olives, drained**
1 **tablespoon chili powder**
1 **teaspoon ground cumin**
½ **cup yellow cornmeal**
½ **cup flour**
1½ **teaspoons baking powder**
½ **cup milk**
1 **egg**
2 **tablespoons vegetable oil**
2 **teaspoons sugar**
½ **cup shredded Monterey Jack or cheddar cheese**

1. In a 9- to 10-inch deep ovenproof skillet or flameproof casserole, cook beef with onion and green pepper over medium high heat, stirring often to break up beef, until beef is browned, about 5 minutes. Drain off excess fat.

2. Stir in tomatoes with their liquid, tomato sauce, corn, olives, chili powder, and cumin. Heat to boiling, reduce heat to low, and simmer 10 minutes.

3. Preheat oven to 400°. Meanwhile in a bowl, combine cornmeal, flour, baking powder, milk, egg, oil, and sugar; mix well. Pour batter over beef mixture in skillet and carefully spread evenly.

4. Bake 18 to 20 minutes, or until cornbread is done. Immediately sprinkle cheese over top. To serve, cut into wedges.

162   BEEF AND BROWN RICE CASSEROLE
Prep: 10 minutes   Cook: 45 minutes   Serves: 6

Perk up jaded appetites with this tasty and easy casserole, a good candidate for potluck fare.

1 **pound lean ground beef**	½ **cup sour cream**
1 **medium onion, chopped**	¼ **cup dry sherry**
1 **(10-ounce) package cut**	¼ **cup water**
Swiss chard, partially	1 **cup quick-cooking brown**
thawed	**rice**
2 **cups broccoli florets**	½ **teaspoon garlic salt**
½ **red bell pepper, chopped**	¼ **teaspoon pepper**
3 **celery ribs, chopped**	1 **cup shredded cheddar**
1 **(10¾-ounce) can condensed**	**cheese**
cream of celery soup,	
undiluted	

1. Preheat oven to 350°. In a large flameproof casserole, cook beef and onion over medium heat, stirring occasionally to break up meat, until beef is browned, about 5 minutes. Drain off fat.

2. Stir in Swiss chard and broccoli and cook 3 minutes.

3. Stir in all remaining ingredients except cheese, mixing well. Increase heat to high and cook, stirring, 2 minutes.

4. Cover and bake 30 to 35 minutes, or until casserole is bubbly and rice is tender. Top with cheese and bake, uncovered, 5 minutes longer to melt cheese.

163   GROUND BEEF VEGETABLE BAKE
Prep: 10 minutes   Cook: 50 minutes   Serves: 5 to 6

Delicious and easy, this is a good way to stretch a pound of ground beef. Substitute other vegetables, if desired.

1 **pound lean ground beef**	1 **(6-ounce) can tomato paste**
1 **medium onion, chopped**	3 **medium zucchini, sliced**
1 **medium green bell pepper,**	3 **cups broccoli florets**
chopped	3 **tablespoons converted rice**
½ **teaspoon garlic powder**	½ **teaspoon salt**
1 **(28-ounce) can cut-up,**	¼ **teaspoon pepper**
peeled tomatoes,	½ **cup shredded cheddar**
undrained	**cheese**

1. Preheat oven to 375°. In a deep 9- or 10-inch ovenproof skillet, cook beef over medium-high heat, stirring occasionally, until browned, about 7 minutes; drain off any fat. Add onion and green pepper and cook, stirring often, until onion is tender, about 3 minutes.

2. Stir in garlic powder, tomatoes with their liquid, and tomato paste. Heat to boiling. Stir in zucchini, broccoli, rice, salt, pepper, and ¼ cup cheese. Heat until mixture bubbles. Reduce heat to low and simmer, uncovered, 10 minutes.

3. Transfer skillet to oven. Bake, uncovered, 30 minutes. Remove from oven and sprinkle remaining ¼ cup cheese over top.

164   CUSTARD-BAKED BEEF AND BLACK-EYED PEAS
Prep: 15 minutes   Cook: 40 minutes   Serves: 4 to 5

For an interesting change of pace, bake a yogurt mixture atop a casserole instead of cheese. Try it on others as well.

1 **pound lean ground beef**	1 **(8-ounce) can tomato sauce**
1 **onion, chopped**	1 **cup plain nonfat yogurt**
4 **zucchini, sliced**	2 **eggs**
½ **red bell pepper, chopped**	2 **teaspoons chopped chives**
½ **teaspoon chili powder**	3 **tablespoons grated**
¼ **teaspoon garlic powder**	**Parmesan cheese**
1 **(10-ounce) package frozen**	
black-eyed peas	

1. Preheat oven to 350°. In a large ovenproof skillet or flameproof casserole, cook beef and onion over medium-high heat, stirring occasionally, until beef is browned, about 5 minutes. Drain off any fat.

2. Stir in zucchini, red pepper, chili powder, and garlic powder. Cook, stirring, until zucchini is crisp-tender, 3 to 5 minutes.

3. Stir in black-eyed peas and tomato sauce. Heat to boiling. Remove from heat. Beat together yogurt, eggs, and chives until well blended. Spread evenly over top of beef mixture. Sprinkle Parmesan cheese evenly over top.

4. Bake, uncovered, 30 minutes, or until topping is set.

---

165 CORNED BEEF, CABBAGE, AND MACARONI HASH

Prep: 10 minutes   Cook: 40 minutes   Serves: 5 to 6

This casserole, made with canned corned beef, is reminiscent of one my brother was fond of during his growing up years. Corned beef from a deli can be substituted for the canned variety, if desired.

8 ounces elbow macaroni
3 cups shredded green cabbage
1 small onion, chopped
1 (12-ounce) can corned beef, chopped
1 (10 ¾-ounce) can condensed cream of mushroom soup
1 cup milk
1 (2-ounce) jar sliced pimientos, chopped
1 tablespoon prepared yellow mustard
¼ teaspoon pepper
1 cup finely diced cheddar cheese cubes (4 ounces)
½ cup dry bread crumbs
1 tablespoon butter, melted

1. Preheat oven to 375°. Fill a large flameproof casserole with salted water. Bring to a boil, add macaroni, and cook 5 minutes. Add cabbage and cook 5 minutes longer. Drain well.

2. Stir in onion, corned beef, undiluted soup, milk, pimiento, mustard, pepper, and diced cheese. Mix well. Spread mixture evenly in casserole, scraping down sides.

3. Toss bread crumbs with butter and sprinkle over top of casserole. Bake, uncovered, 30 minutes, or until hot.

166   TURKEY-EGGPLANT-POTATO BAKE
Prep: 15 minutes   Cook: 55 minutes   Serves: 5 to 6

1 pound lean ground turkey, beef, or lamb
1 medium onion, chopped
1 medium green bell pepper, chopped
2 cups chopped, peeled potatoes (2 medium baking potatoes)
1 medium eggplant (7 x 4½ inches), peeled and chopped
2 garlic cloves, minced

1 (6-ounce) can tomato paste
⅓ cup dry red wine
⅓ cup water
1½ teaspoons chili powder
½ teaspoon ground cumin
1 teaspoon salt
¼ teaspoon pepper
1 cup cottage cheese
1 egg
1 tablespoon chopped parsley
2 tablespoons grated Parmesan cheese

1. In a 10-inch ovenproof skillet or large flameproof casserole, cook turkey and onion over medium-high heat, stirring often, until turkey is no longer pink, about 5 minutes. Drain off any fat.

2. Stir in green pepper, potatoes, eggplant, garlic, tomato paste, red wine, water, chili powder, cumin, salt, and pepper. Heat to boiling. Reduce heat to medium-low. Cover and cook until potatoes and eggplant are tender, about 15 minutes.

3. Preheat oven to 350°. Mix together cottage cheese, egg, and parsley until well blended. Spread evenly over top of eggplant mixture. Sprinkle with Parmesan cheese. Bake about 30 minutes, or until set.

167   TEX-MEX TURKEY STUFFING BAKE
Prep: 10 minutes   Cook: 40 minutes   Serves: 4 to 5

When you have leftover turkey, here's an interesting way to recycle it. You can also use cooked turkey breast available in supermarket meat cases.

1 tablespoon butter
6 scallions, chopped
3 celery ribs, chopped
½ red bell pepper, chopped
1 cup frozen or canned corn kernels
1 (4-ounce) can diced green chiles
¾ teaspoon ground cumin
1 (6-ounce) bag seasoned cornbread stuffing mix (generous 2 cups)

¾ cup water
6 to 8 slices cooked turkey breast
¾ cup mild thick and chunky salsa
½ cup shredded cheddar or Monterey Jack cheese (2 ounces)

1. Preheat oven to 350°. In a 10-inch skillet or large flameproof casserole, melt butter over medium heat. Add scallions, celery, and red pepper. Cook over medium-high heat, stirring often, 2 to 3 minutes, or until soft.

2. Add corn, green chiles, cumin, dry stuffing mix, and water. Mix well. With back of spoon, spread mixture evenly in skillet. Top with turkey slices. Pour salsa over turkey.

3. Cover and bake 30 minutes, or until hot. Remove cover, sprinkle with cheese, and return to oven about 5 minutes to melt cheese.

---

168   CHICKEN POT PIE DELUXE
Prep: 20 minutes   Cook: 1¼ hours   Serves: 4 to 6

This updated version of chicken pot pie is elegant enough for a company meal.

4 tablespoons butter	1 large celery rib, chopped
¼ cup olive oil	1 pound skinless, boneless
½ cup flour	chicken breast halves, cut
2 (14½-ounce) cans chicken	into ½-inch cubes
broth	1 (9- or 10-ounce) package
½ teaspoon thyme	frozen peas and carrots
½ teaspoon ground turmeric	¼ cup chopped parsley
1 teaspoon salt	1 sheet frozen puff pastry
½ teaspoon pepper	(half of a 17¼-ounce
1 large russet potato, peeled	package), cut into ½-inch
and chopped	strips
1 large onion, chopped	

1. Preheat oven to 350°. In a 12-inch round ovenproof skillet 3 inches deep or a flameproof casserole, melt butter with oil over medium-high heat. Add flour and cook, stirring, 1 minute. Whisk in broth and cook, whisking, until sauce boils and thickens, about 2 minutes. Stir in thyme, turmeric, salt, pepper, potato, onion, celery, and chicken.

2. Cover and bake 30 minutes. Remove from oven. Increase oven temperature to 400°.

3. Stir in peas and carrots and parsley. Quickly, but carefully, lay puff pastry strips on top of chicken mixture in lattice-style pattern.

4. Return to oven. Bake, uncovered, 30 minutes longer, or until pastry is puffed and golden.

169   BAKED CHICKEN SUPREME
Prep: 15 minutes   Cook: 50 to 60 minutes   Serves: 4 to 5

This appealing dish would make delicious company fare served with a green salad tossed with fresh fruit.

2 tablespoons butter
5 skinless, boneless chicken
    breast halves
2 cups boiling water
1 cup converted rice
½ teaspoon salt
1 (4-ounce) can diced green
    chiles
1 (16-ounce) package frozen
    corn kernels

1 medium green bell pepper,
    chopped
½ cup mild thick and chunky
    salsa
½ cup sour cream
1½ cups shredded cheddar
    cheese (6 ounces)
    Avocado slices and chopped
    cilantro, for garnish

1. In a deep 9- or 10-inch ovenproof skillet, melt butter over medium heat. Add chicken breasts (in two batches, if necessary) and cook on both sides until golden, 10 to 12 minutes total. Remove to a plate.

2. Add water, rice, and salt to skillet. Heat to boiling, stirring occasionally. Stir in green chiles, corn, and green pepper. Reduce heat to low, cover, and simmer 20 to 25 minutes, until rice is tender.

3. Preheat oven to 375°. Mix salsa, sour cream, and 1 cup cheese. Spoon half the mixture over rice. Arrange chicken on top. Cover with remaining salsa mixture.

4. Sprinkle with remaining ½ cup cheese. Bake, uncovered, 15 to 20 minutes, or until hot throughout. Garnish each serving with sliced avocado and cilantro.

170   APRICOT-ORANGE PORK TENDERLOIN
Prep: 20 minutes   Cook: 55 minutes   Serves: 4

1 large navel orange
1 tablespoon peanut oil
1½ pounds pork tenderloin (2
    pieces, each 6 to 8 inches
    long)
1 medium green bell pepper,
    chopped
1 medium onion, chopped
3 garlic cloves, minced

½ teaspoon ground ginger
1 (6.25-ounce) package quick-
    cooking long-grain and
    wild rice mix
1 (17-ounce) can apricot halves
    packed in heavy syrup
1 (6-ounce) package frozen
    pea pods

1. Preheat oven to 350°. Grate zest from orange and set aside. Remove and discard white pith. Separate orange into segments and reserve.

2. In a 3-quart flameproof casserole, heat peanut oil over medium-high heat until hot. Add pork tenderloins and cook, turning, until browned, 2 to 3 minutes. Remove and set aside.

3. Add green pepper and onion to same casserole and cook over medium-high heat, stirring, until onion is softened but not browned, about 2 minutes. Stir in garlic, ginger, orange zest, and rice and seasonings from mix. Reduce heat to low. Drain syrup from apricots into a 2-cup measure. Add enough water to measure 2 cups. Stir into rice mixture. Place tenderloins on top of rice mixture.

4. Cover and bake 45 minutes, or until pork is cooked through. Add pea pods, orange segments, and apricot halves; do not mix in. Bake, uncovered, 5 minutes longer, or until pea pods are heated through. To serve, with sharp knife, slice pork thin on the diagonal. Serve on rice with apricots and oranges on top.

171 CHINESE PORK CASSEROLE
Prep: 30 minutes   Cook: 1¼ hours   Serves: 6 to 8

Brown rice, pork, and vegetables team together in this Chinese-inspired casserole.

2 tablespoons peanut oil	½ pound Napa cabbage, shredded (about ½ head)
1½ pounds boneless pork shoulder, cut into 1-inch cubes	1 (14½-ounce) can chicken broth
1 medium red bell pepper, cut into ½-inch strips	1¾ cups quick-cooking brown rice
1 medium yellow bell pepper, cut into ½-inch strips	1 (8-ounce) can sliced water chestnuts, drained
2 carrots, peeled and cut into thin strips	3 tablespoons soy sauce
6 dried shiitake mushrooms, soaked, drained, and cut into thin strips	1 tablespoon Asian sesame oil
	1 (6-ounce) package frozen Chinese pea pods
	5 scallions, thinly sliced

1. Preheat oven to 350°. In a large flameproof casserole, heat peanut oil over high heat. Add pork and cook, stirring often, until browned, about 5 minutes.

2. Add red and yellow peppers and carrots and cook, stirring often, 2 minutes. Stir in mushrooms, cabbage, broth, rice, water chestnuts, soy sauce, and sesame oil.

3. Cover and bake 1 hour. Stir in frozen pea pods, cover, and let stand 5 minutes. Garnish with scallions.

172 HASH BROWN AND EGG BRUNCH CASSEROLE
Prep: 10 minutes   Cook: 35 minutes   Serves: 4 to 5

Here's the way to end up with hash browns and eggs in a single dish for a trouble-free morning or evening offering.

4 tablespoons butter	8 eggs
1 medium onion, chopped	½ cup heavy cream
1 medium red bell pepper, chopped	1 (4-ounce) can diced green chiles
1 medium green bell pepper, chopped	½ teaspoon salt
1 (24-ounce) package frozen hash brown potatoes, thawed	¼ teaspoon pepper
	2 cups shredded Monterey Jack or cheddar cheese (8 ounces)

1. Preheat oven to 350°. In a deep 9-inch or 10-inch ovenproof skillet, melt butter over medium heat. Add onion and peppers and cook until onion is softened, about 3 minutes.

2. Add potatoes and cook, covered, over medium heat 5 minutes.

3. Beat together eggs and cream; stir in chiles, salt, and pepper. Pour evenly over potato mixture. Sprinkle cheese evenly over top.

4. Cover and bake 10 minutes. Uncover and continue baking 15 to 17 minutes, until almost set in center.

173 MUSHROOM-BARLEY VEGETABLE BAKE
Prep: 10 minutes   Cook: 65 minutes   Serves: 4

This versatile dish can be served as an entrée with or without meat.

3 tablespoons butter	2 cups boiling water
¾ cup sliced or slivered almonds	2 (.19-ounce) packets instant vegetable broth and seasoning mix
1 onion, chopped	½ cup dark raisins
½ pound fresh mushrooms, quartered	2 cups chopped fresh kale
1 cup pearl barley	1½ cups frozen peas and carrots

1. Preheat oven to 350°. In a deep 9-inch or 10-inch ovenproof skillet, melt 1 tablespoon butter over medium heat. Add almonds and cook, stirring, over medium heat until golden, about 2 minutes. Remove to a dish and set aside.

2. Melt remaining 2 tablespoons butter in skillet. Add onion, mushrooms, and barley. Cook, stirring often, over medium heat, until barley is golden brown, about 5 minutes.

3. Stir in 1 cup boiling water and contents of 1 broth packet. Cover and bake 20 minutes.

4. Uncover and stir in remaining 1 cup boiling water, remaining broth packet, raisins, almonds, and kale. Cover and bake 25 to 30 minutes longer.

5. Remove from oven. Stir in peas and carrots. Cover and let stand 10 minutes before serving.

---

174   CHEDDAR NOODLE CASSEROLE

Prep: 10 minutes   Cook: 35 to 40 minutes   Serves: 5 to 6

This is an attractive and delicious casserole that's good for a special buffet or potluck offering.

1 (9-ounce) package fresh spinach linguine or other spinach noodles
1 (10 ¾-ounce) can condensed cream of mushroom soup
¾ cup milk
2 cups grated cheddar cheese (½ pound)
¼ teaspoon garlic powder
3 tablespoons dry sherry
½ red bell pepper, chopped, or 1 (2-ounce) jar sliced pimientos, chopped

1 (8-ounce) can sliced water chestnuts, drained
1 (4-ounce) can mushroom stems and pieces, drained
2 cups chopped smoked turkey breast or cooked chicken
1 cup blanched slivered almonds (4 ounces)

1. Fill a large ovenproof skillet or flameproof casserole with salted water. Bring to a boil, add pasta, and cook until almost tender, 2 to 3 minutes. Drain well.

2. Preheat oven to 350°. Add undiluted soup, milk, and cheese to pasta in casserole and cook over low heat, stirring often, until cheese melts, about 2 minutes.

3. Stir in garlic powder, sherry, red pepper, water chestnuts, mushrooms, smoked turkey, and ⅓ cup almonds. Mix to blend well. Scrape down sides of pan and spread mixture out evenly. Sprinkle top with remaining ⅔ cup almonds.

4. Bake, uncovered, 30 to 35 minutes, until bubbly around edges and hot throughout.

175   SPINACH NOODLE BAKE
Prep: 10 minutes   Cook: 40 minutes   Serves: 4 to 5

Here's a meatless noodle dish that is just plain delicious.

1 (7-ounce) package egg
   noodle bows
1 medium onion, chopped
¼ teaspoon garlic powder
¼ teaspoon pepper
2 (10-ounce) packages frozen
   chopped spinach, thawed

1 (10 ¾-ounce) can condensed
   cream of celery soup
3 tablespoons sour cream
1 cup shredded sharp cheddar
   cheese (4 ounces)

1. Preheat oven to 350°. Fill a deep 9-inch ovenproof skillet or a large flame-proof casserole with salted water and bring to a boil. Add noodles and cook 10 to 12 minutes, or until tender. Drain off water.

2. Stir in onion, garlic powder, pepper, undrained spinach, undiluted soup, sour cream, and ½ cup cheese. Mix thoroughly.

3. Bake, uncovered, 20 minutes. Sprinkle with remaining ½ cup cheese and bake 10 minutes longer, until cheese is melted.

176   ZUCCHINI AND CHEESE QUICHE
Prep: 10 minutes   Cook: 50 minutes   Serves: 4 to 5

This is a good recipe to give a whirl when you have an abundant supply of zucchini on hand. It's a satisfying supper offering with a fruit salad.

2 tablespoons butter
2 cups chopped zucchini
2 scallions, chopped
1 (4-ounce) can diced green
   chiles
1 large tomato, chopped
1½ cups shredded cheddar
   cheese (6 ounces)

1½ cups shredded Monterey
   Jack cheese (6 ounces)
6 eggs
⅓ cup milk
¼ teaspoon garlic salt
⅛ teaspoon pepper

1. Preheat oven to 350°. Heat butter in a 9-inch ovenproof skillet over medium heat until melted. Add zucchini and scallions and cook, stirring, until crisp-tender, about 5 minutes. Remove from heat and let cool 5 to 10 minutes.

2. Stir in green chiles and tomato, then cheeses.

3. In a medium bowl, beat together eggs, milk, garlic salt, and pepper until well mixed. Pour over cheese mixture. Bake 40 to 45 minutes, until set in center.

Chapter 5

Casseroles and Bakes

Once a haven for lonely leftovers, casseroles—updated and modernized—have been staging a comeback in the past few years. We've included a wealth of styles and flavors in this chapter, with many recipes built on fresh foods with good nutrition in mind. The only criteria was the style of cooking—oven baking in an earthenware, porcelain, or heatproof glass casserole or baking dish. Because of the nature of casseroles and bakes—you'll find many terrific brunch choices here—crustless quiches, stratas, and savory puffs.

Even lasagne and ravioli are possible one-dish meals when you rely on the recipes here—no precooking of the pasta necessary. Remember, many casseroles make good choices to tote when you're asked to bring a meal in a dish to a potluck supper.

Glazed Chicken Bake is a good bet for a casual company gathering. Try Pineapple-Ham Bean Bake for a weeknight meal. Salmon and Potato Scallop takes advantage of scalloped potato mix, while Broccoli Soufflé Bake is a great way to utilize diced cooked chicken. And who wouldn't enjoy Chicken and Black Bean Enchiladas or Lasagne Florentine?

Not only are casseroles easy to make and simple to serve, but they're time-savers that usually require no last-minute preparation. And many can be baked in advance and reheated just before serving.

177   CHINESE CHICKEN STRATA
Prep: 15 minutes   Cook: 40 to 45 minutes   Serves: 5 to 6

Here's an easy way to make dinner in a dish well in advance. Chinese chicken salad was the inspiration for this tasty rendition filled with chicken, red pepper, water chestnuts, and soy sauce.

3 cups diced cooked chicken
3 tablespoons reduced-sodium soy sauce
1½ tablespoons rice vinegar
1½ tablespoons Asian sesame oil
1 teaspoon chili paste with garlic
1¾ teaspoons dry mustard
4 scallions, chopped
1 medium red bell pepper, chopped

1 (8-ounce) can sliced water chestnuts, well drained
6 slices buttermilk or white bread, crusts removed, cut into 1-inch cubes
2 cups mild cheddar cheese, shredded (½ pound)
3 eggs
2 cups milk

1. In a medium bowl, combine diced chicken, soy sauce, vinegar, sesame oil, chili paste with garlic, 1 teaspoon dry mustard, scallions, red pepper, and water chestnuts. Mix well and set aside.

2. Turn half the bread cubes into a buttered 11 × 7-inch baking dish. Sprinkle with half the cheese. Distribute half the chicken mixture over cheese. Cover with remaining bread cubes and remaining chicken mixture. Top with remaining cheese.

3. Beat together eggs, milk, and remaining ¾ teaspoon dry mustard until blended. Pour evenly over casserole. Cover with plastic wrap. Refrigerate several hours, or overnight.

4. Preheat oven to 350°. Bake, uncovered, 40 to 45 minutes, until top is golden and center is set. Let cool 5 minutes, then cut into squares or rectangles to serve.

178 GLAZED CHICKEN BAKE
Prep: 15 minutes   Cook: 1½ hours   Serves: 5 to 6

You won't believe the combination of ingredients—cranberry sauce, French dressing, and onion soup mix—that makes this dish so delicious.

1½ cups converted rice
2 cups boiling water
3 scallions, chopped
1 (16-ounce) can whole berry cranberry sauce
1 (8-ounce) bottle French dressing
1 (1.2-ounce) envelope dry onion soup mix
6 bone-in chicken breast halves, skinned
1 (10-ounce) package frozen mixed vegetables

1. Preheat oven to 350°. In bottom of a 9 × 13-inch baking dish, combine rice, boiling water, and scallions. Mix well.

2. In a medium bowl, combine cranberry sauce, French dressing, and dry soup. Mix to blend well. Using about one third of mixture, place several spoonfuls evenly over rice mixture.

3. Arrange chicken breasts evenly on top. Spoon remaining cranberry mixture over and around chicken breasts, spreading evenly.

4. Cover with foil. Bake 1¼ hours. Remove foil, sprinkle vegetables all around chicken, and carefully mix into rice. Bake 15 minutes longer, or until vegetables are hot and cooked through.

179 CHICKEN ENCHILADA CASSEROLE
Prep: 15 minutes   Cook: 35 minutes   Serves: 6

Serve this tasty dish topped with guacamole and encircle individual servings with shredded lettuce, if desired.

9 (7- or 8-inch) corn tortillas
1 (28-ounce) can crushed tomatoes with added puree
2 cups shredded cooked chicken
4 scallions, chopped
1 (7-ounce) can diced green chiles
1 (2.2-ounce) can sliced ripe olives, drained
1½ cups sour cream
2 cups shredded cheddar cheese (8 ounces)

1. Preheat oven to 350°. In a 12 × 8-inch baking dish, place 3 tortillas, overlapping slightly, as necessary. Layer one third of tomatoes, chicken, scallions, chiles, olives, sour cream, and cheese over tortillas.

2. Cover with another 3 tortillas and layer half of remaining tomatoes, chicken, scallions, chilies, olives, sour cream, and cheese. Then repeat layers again, ending with tomatoes and cheese.

3. Bake, uncovered, about 35 minutes, or until bubbly and heated through.

180 APRICOT-GLAZED CHICKEN
Prep: 10 minutes   Cook: 1½ hours   Serves: 4 to 5

Once you've whipped together this creation, the oven does the rest. This would be an appealing company offering for a casual gathering when you want a fuss-free entrée.

1 medium leek (white and tender green), washed well and chopped
1 cup converted rice
⅓ cup wild rice
1 pound carrots, peeled, halved lengthwise, and cut into 2-inch lengths
1 teaspoon salt
½ teaspoon pepper

1¾ cups boiling water
½ cup apricot preserves
½ cup bottled Russian dressing
½ envelope (about 2 generous tablespoons) dry onion soup mix
6 bone-in chicken breast halves, skinned

1. Preheat oven to 350°. In bottom of a 9 × 13-inch baking dish, sprinkle leek, converted and wild rice, and carrots. Season with salt and pepper. Pour water evenly over all.

2. In a small bowl, combine apricot preserves, Russian dressing, and dry soup mix. Stir to blend well.

3. Place chicken on top of rice mixture. Spread dressing mixture evenly over chicken, placing a little bit between chicken pieces.

4. Cover with foil. Bake 1¼ hours. Uncover and bake 15 to 20 minutes longer, or until rice is tender and most or all liquid is absorbed.

---

181 CHICKEN AND BLACK BEAN ENCHILADAS
Prep: 20 minutes   Cook: 30 minutes   Serves: 6

Stuff flour tortillas with cut-up cooked chicken (or turkey) and black beans for this updated enchilada. Whip together a sauce with tomato puree, a fresh diced tomato, and chili powder. Or simply use canned enchilada sauce.

1 (16-ounce) can tomato puree
3 tablespoons water
1 large tomato, chopped
2 teaspoons chili powder
2 cups cut-up cooked chicken or turkey
½ cup sour cream
1 (4-ounce) can diced green chiles

1 (16-ounce) can black beans, rinsed and well drained
1¼ cups shredded cheddar cheese (5 ounces)
10 (8-inch) flour tortillas (18-ounce package)
3 scallions, chopped

1. Preheat oven to 350°. Combine tomato puree, water, tomato, and chili powder. Spoon about one third of mixture over bottom of a 9 × 13-inch baking dish. Set aside.

2. In a medium bowl, mix together chicken, sour cream, green chiles, black beans, and ¾ cup cheese. Place a generous ¼ cup bean mixture close to one edge of each tortilla, spreading out the length of tortilla. Roll up tightly, jelly-roll fashion.

3. Place enchiladas, seam sides down, very close together atop sauce in baking dish. Spoon remaining sauce evenly over enchiladas.

4. Bake, uncovered, 25 minutes. Sprinkle top with remaining ½ cup cheese, return to oven, and bake 5 minutes longer, until cheese melts and enchiladas are hot. Garnish with scallions. Serve with additional sour cream and guacamole on the side, if desired.

---

182 TURKEY BREAST WITH GRAPEFRUIT
Prep: 30 minutes   Cook: 1½ hours   Serves: 4 to 6

Grapefruit lends refreshing flavor to this dish.

1 **(16-ounce) can grapefruit segments**
2 **carrots, peeled and cut into thin 2-inch-long sticks**
2 **celery ribs, cut into thin 2-inch-long sticks**
6 **scallions, cut into thin 2-inch-long pieces**
¼ **cup chopped fresh cilantro or parsley**
3 **garlic cloves, minced**
1 **large baking potato (¾ pound), peeled and cut into thin 2-inch-long pieces**

1 **(6.25-ounce) package fast-cooking long-grain and wild rice mix**
1 **(2½-pound) skinless, boneless turkey breast half**
1 **tablespoon Dijon mustard**
1 **tablespoon soy sauce**
2 **tablespoons orange marmalade**
½ **teaspoon pepper**

1. Preheat oven to 350°. Drain juice from grapefruit into a 2-cup measure. Add enough water to make 1½ cups; set aside.

2. In a 4- or 5-quart, 3-inch deep casserole dish with lid, mix together carrots, celery, scallions, cilantro, garlic, potato, reserved grapefruit liquid, and rice and seasonings from mix. Lay turkey breast, most attractive side up, on top of rice mixture.

3. Mix together mustard, soy sauce, marmalade, and pepper. Carefully pour over turkey breast (some sauce will drip down into vegetables). Roast, uncovered, 1 hour.

4. Cover and roast 30 minutes longer, or until internal temperature of turkey reaches 170°. Serve turkey, sliced, on a bed of rice, topped with grapefruit segments.

183   LEFTOVER TURKEY BAKE

Prep: 10 minutes   Cook: 40 to 45 minutes   Serves: 6

This casserole is made-to-order for using leftover cooked turkey and/or leftover rice. You can also use turkey ham, which is already cooked and can be found in supermarket meat sections.

3   cups cooked rice
3   cups frozen French-cut
    green beans
1   (2-ounce) jar sliced
    pimientos, drained
1   large onion, chopped
1   medium green bell pepper,
    chopped

2   cups diced cooked turkey or
    turkey ham
1   (10¾-ounce) can cream of
    mushroom soup
½   cup water or milk
2   tablespoons dry sherry
½   cup sliced or slivered
    blanched almonds

1. Preheat oven to 350°. In a 2½-quart casserole, combine rice, green beans, pimientos, onion, and green pepper; mix well. Spread evenly in dish.

2. Sprinkle turkey over rice mixture in casserole. Mix soup with water and sherry and pour over all. Sprinkle almonds on top.

3. Bake casserole, uncovered, 40 to 45 minutes, or until bubbling and lightly browned.

TUNA BAKE

Substitute 2 or 3 (6½- or 7-ounce) cans solid white tuna packed in water, drained, for turkey. Replace almonds with ½ cup cashews.

184   FRUITED TURKEY BREAST

Prep: 10 minutes   Cook: 1¾ hours   Serves: 4 to 5

This is a wonderful way to prepare turkey year-round, but it would be particularly nice for a small gathering on Thanksgiving, too.

1   (3-pound) turkey breast half
½   teaspoon thyme
½   teaspoon rosemary
1   large onion, chopped
1   large green bell pepper,
    chopped
3   carrots, peeled and chopped
1   (8-ounce) package dried
    mixed fruit (prunes,
    pears, apples, and
    apricots), coarsely
    chopped

1   sweet potato, peeled and
    chopped
1   (8-ounce) can unsweetened
    pineapple chunks, juice
    reserved
1   tablespoon brown sugar
2   tablespoons ketchup
½   cup dry red wine

1. Preheat oven to 450°. Place turkey breast, skin side up, in a 13 × 9-inch or 13 × 10-inch casserole dish or baking pan. Sprinkle turkey breast with thyme and rosemary. Roast, uncovered, 25 minutes. Remove from oven. Drain off and discard any fat and juices.

2. Reduce oven temperature to 350°. Arrange onion, green pepper, carrots, dried fruit, sweet potato, and pineapple chunks around turkey.

3. Mix together reserved pineapple juice, brown sugar, ketchup, and red wine. Pour over and around turkey. Cover pan loosely with foil. Return to oven and bake 1 hour longer.

4. Remove foil and continue baking 20 to 30 minutes, basting occasionally with pan juices, until sauce is thickened and turkey is cooked through.

---

185 TURKEY AND HASH BROWN PIE
Prep: 15 minutes   Cook: 45 minutes   Serves: 6

This is downright good old-fashioned comfort food, updated with ground turkey instead of ground beef, in a single dish.

1½ **pounds ground turkey**	½ **teaspoon garlic powder**
1 **cup shredded carrots**	¾ **teaspoon salt**
(2 carrots)	¼ **teaspoon pepper**
3 **scallions, chopped**	16 **ounces frozen hash brown**
1 **celery rib, chopped**	**potatoes, thawed**
¾ **cup Italian seasoned bread**	2 **tablespoons butter, melted**
crumbs	¾ **cup shredded cheddar**
1 **egg**	**cheese**
1 **tablespoon Worcestershire**	
sauce	

1. Preheat oven to 350°. In a large bowl, combine turkey, carrots, scallions, celery, bread crumbs, egg, Worcestershire sauce, garlic powder, salt, and pepper. Mix to blend well.

2. Form a shell by spreading turkey mixture evenly in bottom and up sides of 10-inch pie dish.

3. Place potatoes in turkey shell and drizzle with melted butter.

4. Bake 40 minutes, or until turkey is cooked through. Top with cheese and bake 5 minutes longer, or until cheese melts.

186   TURKEY-RICE BAKE
Prep: 10 minutes   Cook: 1 hour   Serves: 4 to 5

Mix and bake all in the same dish, thanks to a package of long-grain and wild rice mix.

1 (6-ounce) package long-grain and wild rice mix
1½ cups boiling water
2 cups frozen green beans
2 cups diced cooked leftover turkey or hickory-smoked turkey breast
1 (4-ounce) can mushroom stems and pieces, drained

¼ cup chopped roasted red pepper or pimiento
½ cup coarsely chopped pimiento-stuffed green olives
1 cup shredded Fontina cheese

1. Preheat oven to 375°. In a 2-quart casserole or 11 × 7-inch baking dish, combine rice and seasonings from rice mix with boiling water. Mix well.

2. Stir in green beans, turkey, mushrooms, roasted red pepper, and olives. Cover dish with foil. Bake 30 minutes. Uncover dish and stir all ingredients to mix well. Cover and bake 20 minutes longer.

3. Uncover casserole and bake 5 minutes, or until all liquid is absorbed. Top with cheese and bake 5 minutes longer, or until cheese melts.

187   TURKEY STUFFED PEPPERS
Prep: 15 minutes   Cook: 1¼ hours   Serves: 4

For a change of pace, stuff green bell peppers with ground turkey rather than ground beef. With this recipe variation, you can stuff peppers in a hurry and let the oven do the rest. There's no need to cook the meat and rice or blanch the peppers in advance of baking.

4 large green bell peppers
½ pound ground turkey
½ onion, chopped
1 celery rib, chopped
1 teaspoon celery seeds
⅛ teaspoon pepper

½ cup converted rice
1 (15-ounce) can tomato sauce
¾ cup shredded cheddar cheese
½ cup Burgundy or other dry red wine

1. Preheat oven to 400°. Slice tops off peppers and remove seeds. Stand peppers up in a deep 3-quart baking dish.

2. Combine uncooked turkey, onion, celery, celery seeds, pepper, and rice; mix well. Mix in ½ cup tomato sauce and ½ cup cheese.

3. Stuff peppers with turkey mixture, dividing evenly.

4. Mix remaining tomato sauce, remaining ¼ cup cheese, and wine. Pour over and around peppers. Cover dish with foil.

5. Bake 45 minutes. Remove cover from casserole, reduce oven temperature to 375°, and continue baking 30 minutes, or until rice is tender, basting peppers a few times with sauce.

188 TURKEY TORTILLA BAKE
Prep: 10 minutes   Cook: 1 hour 5 minutes   Serves: 6

This is reminiscent of a meat loaf but is layered between tortillas and has Tex-Mex flavors with salsa and green chiles.

1 **pound ground turkey**
2 **cups shredded cheddar cheese (8 ounces)**
2 **scallions, chopped**
1 **(12-ounce) jar mild green chili salsa**
1 **(2.2-ounce) can sliced ripe olives, drained**

1 **(4-ounce) can diced green chiles**
6 **(12-inch) flour tortillas**
1 **tomato, chopped (½ cup)**
Optional accompaniments: Sour cream and guacamole

1. Preheat oven to 400°. Combine turkey, 1 cup cheese, scallions, 1 cup salsa, olives, and green chiles; mix well.

2. Line a 12 × 8-inch rectangular baking dish with 2 tortillas, extending part way up sides of dish. Spread half the turkey mixture over tortillas. Top with 2 more tortillas, torn to fit atop turkey mixture.

3. Top with remaining turkey mixture, then remaining 2 tortillas. Sprinkle top with remaining 1 cup cheese, remaining salsa, and tomatoes.

4. Cover with foil. Bake 35 minutes. Remove foil and continue baking 30 minutes longer, or until turkey is cooked through. To serve, cut into squares and top with sour cream and guacamole, if desired.

189 PINEAPPLE-HAM BEAN BAKE
Prep: 10 minutes   Cook: 35 minutes   Serves: 4 to 5

This quick-to-fix dish is a great way to use leftover baked ham.

1 **medium onion, chopped**
1 **(20-ounce) can unsweetened pineapple chunks, drained**
½ **pound baked ham, chopped (about 2 cups)**
1 **(15-ounce) can cooked dry butter beans, drained**

2 **(15½-ounce) cans Texas-style barbecue beans, undrained**
1 **tablespoon white wine vinegar**
¼ **teaspoon dry mustard, or 2 teaspoons prepared yellow mustard**

1. Preheat oven to 375°. In a shallow 2½-quart casserole, combine onion, pineapple chunks, ham, butter beans, barbecue beans with their liquid, wine vinegar, and mustard. Mix thoroughly until well combined.

2. Bake, uncovered, 35 minutes, until very hot and bubbly.

190   SCALLOPED HAM, POTATOES, AND LEEKS
Prep: 15 minutes   Cook: 1¼ hours   Serves: 6

This is an old-fashioned comfort food, updated and turned into a one-dish meal with the addition of ham. Keep this in mind for a tasty brunch selection.

6 cups sliced, peeled russet potatoes (about 5 large)	4½ tablespoons flour
1 large leek (white and tender green), washed well and chopped	12 ounces fully cooked ham slices
1 (2-ounce) jar sliced pimientos, drained	¼ teaspoon salt
	¼ teaspoon pepper
	1¾ cups milk
	2 tablespoons butter

1. Preheat oven to 350°. Arrange one third of potatoes in a greased 2½-quart oval casserole dish. Sprinkle with a third each of leeks and pimientos, then 1½ tablespoons flour. Add a layer of half the ham slices.

2. Add half of remaining potatoes, leeks, and pimientos. Top with remaining ham slices and 1½ tablespoons flour.

3. Top with a final layer of potato slices, sprinkle with remaining 1½ tablespoons flour, remaining leeks, pimientos, and salt and pepper. Pour milk over all. Dot with butter.

4. Cover and bake 35 minutes. Uncover and bake 30 to 35 minutes longer, or until potatoes are tender and liquid is reduced to desired consistency. Let stand 5 minutes before serving.

---

191   EASY PORK CHOP DINNER
Prep: 10 minutes   Cook: 2 hours   Serves: 6

Simply layer all ingredients in a rectangular dish and let the oven do the rest.

1 quart sauerkraut, rinsed and well drained	1 (14½-ounce) can peeled tomatoes, undrained and cut up
6 (¾-inch-thick) boneless pork chops (about 1½ pounds total), trimmed of excess fat	½ green bell pepper, chopped
	1 tablespoon caraway seeds
2 medium onions, sliced	¼ teaspon salt
5 medium potatoes, peeled and cut into ½-inch-thick rounds	⅛ teaspoon pepper

1. Preheat oven to 350°. In a 9 × 13-inch glass baking dish, layer ingredients as follows: sauerkraut, pork chops, onion slices, potato rounds, and tomatoes with their liquid. Sprinkle with green pepper and caraway seeds. Season with salt and pepper.

2. Cover with foil. Bake 1½ hours. Remove foil and continue baking, uncovered, ½ hour longer.

192 BAKED REUBEN CASSEROLE
Prep: 15 minutes   Cook: 40 minutes   Serves: 6

All of the flavors in a Reuben sandwich are combined in this casserole dish. The meat choice is yours: either turkey ham or corned beef.

6 slices rye bread, preferably with dill
2 tablespoons Russian or Thousand Island dressing
6 ounces thinly sliced turkey ham or corned beef
1½ cups rinsed and well-drained sauerkraut

2 dill pickles, chopped
½ teaspoon caraway seeds
2 cups shredded Swiss cheese (8 ounces)
3 eggs
1½ cups milk
1 tablespoon prepared yellow mustard

1. Butter an 11 × 7-inch baking dish. Line bottom of dish with 3 bread slices, cutting as necessary to fit.

2. Spread 1 tablespoon dressing over bread. Cover with half the ham, then top with half the sauerkraut, half the pickles, and ¼ teaspoon caraway seeds. Sprinkle evenly with half the cheese. Cover with remaining 3 bread slices cut to fit dish and spread with remaining 1 tablespoon dressing. Repeat layers as above.

3. With a whisk, beat together eggs, milk, and mustard until well mixed. Pour over casserole. Let stand while oven is heating.

4. Preheat oven to 350°. Bake casserole 40 minutes, or until light golden and set in center.

193 GREEN CHILE AND RICE CASSEROLE
Prep: 5 minutes   Cook: 30 to 35 minutes   Serves: 4 to 5

A good meatless main dish and a good way to use leftover rice. Serve with a tossed green salad.

3 cups cooked rice
1½ cups low-fat cottage cheese
⅓ cup milk
1 (4-ounce) can diced green chiles
1 (12-ounce) can corn kernels, drained

1½ cups shredded cheddar cheese (6 ounces)
⅓ cup chopped roasted red peppers or pimiento
¼ cup grated Parmesan cheese

1. Preheat oven to 350°. In a 2-quart casserole, combine rice, cottage cheese, milk, chiles, corn, cheddar cheese, and red peppers. Mix until well blended.

2. Sprinkle Parmesan cheese over top. Bake casserole 30 to 35 minutes.

194   MEXICAN PUMPKIN
Prep: 20 minutes   Cook: 2½ hours   Serves: 6

This is a good way to use a leftover uncarved Halloween pumpkin. Pumpkins vary in moisture content. Some pumpkins will sag during baking and juices will run into bottom of pan; others will remain firm, allowing them to be presented and used as serving containers at the table.

1 (10-pound) pumpkin
1 (11-ounce) can Mexicorn (whole kernel corn with red and green peppers), drained
1 (4-ounce) can diced green chiles
1 (8¾-ounce) can garbanzo beans (chick-peas), drained
1 (15-ounce) can pinto beans, drained
1 (3¼-ounce) can pitted ripe olives, drained

1 (14½-ounce) can cut-up, peeled tomatoes, undrained
1 (6-ounce) can tomato paste
1 teaspoon minced jalepeño pepper
1 teaspoon chili powder
½ teaspoon ground cumin
½ teaspoon dried oregano
¼ teaspoon salt
2½ pounds ground turkey
6 scallions, sliced
1 cup sour cream

1. Preheat oven to 325°. Cut off top of pumpkin, decoratively if desired, and remove. Clean off top and clean out inside of pumpkin, scraping to remove all strings and seeds.

2. Inside pumpkin, mix together Mexicorn, chiles, garbanzo beans, pinto beans, olives, tomatoes with their liquid, tomato paste, jalepeño, chili powder, cumin, oregano, and salt. Add ground turkey crumbled into pieces and mix well. Replace top on pumpkin. Place pumpkin in a shallow 9 × 13-inch baking pan. Bake 1 hour.

3. Remove pumpkin top, stir ingredients inside pumpkin, and bake 1 hour. Stir ingredients again and bake 30 minutes, or until tender but not falling apart and turkey is cooked through. As the meat mixture is scooped out to serve, scoop out some of the cooked pumpkin also. Serve topped with a sprinkling of scallions and a dollop of sour cream.

195   CHILES RELLENOS CORN CASSEROLE
Prep: 10 minutes   Cook: 40 to 45 minutes   Serves: 6

Serve this meatless entrée topped with lettuce, salsa, guacamole, and sour cream, or accompany with a tossed green or fresh fruit salad.

¾ cup milk
2 eggs
⅓ cup flour
1 cup chopped fresh tomatoes
1 (7-ounce) can diced green chiles
1 cup drained canned corn

1½ cups shredded cheddar cheese (6 ounces)
1½ cups shredded Monterey Jack cheese (6 ounces)
Optional accompaniments: Shredded lettuce, salsa, guacamole, sour cream

1. Preheat oven to 375°. In a deep 1½-quart casserole, whisk together milk, eggs, and flour until smooth. Stir in all remaining ingredients; mix well.

2. Bake casserole 40 to 45 minutes, or until set in center. Serve warm topped with shredded lettuce, salsa, guacamole, and sour cream, if desired.

196   BROCCOLI SOUFFLE BAKE
Prep: 15 minutes   Cook: 35 to 45 minutes   Serves: 8 to 10

This recipe, adapted from one a friend shared, is a wonderful way to use leftover cooked chicken or turkey. It's a good and easy choice for a potluck contribution, too.

2 (1-pound) packages frozen chopped broccoli, thawed and drained
2 or 3 cups leftover diced (½-inch cubes) cooked chicken or turkey
1 cup reduced-calorie mayonnaise
2 eggs
1 (10¾-ounce) can condensed cream of mushroom soup

¼ teaspoon pepper
2 cups shredded sharp cheddar cheese (8 ounces)
1½ cups finely crushed Ritz crackers
4 tablespoons butter or margarine, melted
½ teaspoon garlic powder

1. Preheat oven to 350°. Line a 9 × 13-inch baking dish evenly with broccoli. Sprinkle chicken over broccoli.

2. In a medium bowl, mix together mayonnaise, eggs, undiluted soup, pepper, and cheese until thoroughly combined. Pour over chicken and broccoli.

3. In a medium bowl, mix together thoroughly cracker crumbs, melted butter, and garlic powder. Sprinkle evenly over top.

4. Bake, uncovered, 35 to 45 minutes, or until top is golden and casserole is hot and bubbly.

197 CRAZY VEGETABLE PIE
Prep: 10 minutes   Cook: 30 minutes   Serves: 6

This is an easy brunch or supper offering. Accompany with seasonal fresh fruits.

1 cup chopped tomatoes	1½ cups milk
1 cup chopped zucchini	¾ cup buttermilk baking mix,
1 cup chopped yellow	such as Bisquick
crookneck squash	3 eggs
1 cup (packed) chopped fresh	1 teaspoon Worcestershire
spinach	sauce
2 scallions, chopped	2 teaspoons Dijon mustard
¼ cup grated Parmesan cheese	

1. Preheat oven to 400°. Scatter tomatoes, zucchini, squash, spinach, scallions, and cheese over bottom of a greased 10-inch quiche dish or pie plate.

2. In a medium bowl, whisk together milk, buttermilk baking mix, eggs, Worcestershire, and mustard until smooth. Pour over vegetables.

3. Bake about 30 minutes, or until knife inserted in center comes out clean. Let pie stand 5 minutes before serving.

198 BAKED LENTILS AND VEGETABLES WITH CHEDDAR CHEESE
Prep: 15 minutes   Cook: 1 hour 10 minutes   Serves: 6

This is a substantial and delightful meatless main dish. The recipe was adapted from one a colleague shared several years ago.

2 cups lentils, rinsed and	1 (14½-ounce) can cut-up,
picked over	peeled tomatoes,
2¼ cups hot water	undrained
2 medium onions, chopped	4 carrots, peeled and chopped
2 garlic cloves, minced	½ pound fresh green beans,
2 bay leaves	cut into 1-inch pieces
½ teaspoon salt	3 tablespoons chopped
¼ teaspoon pepper	parsley
¼ teaspoon marjoram	2 cups shredded sharp
¼ teaspoon sage	cheddar cheese (8 ounces)

1. Preheat oven to 375°. In a 9 × 13-inch baking dish or shallow 3½- or 4-quart oval casserole, combine lentils, water, onions, garlic, bay leaves, salt, pepper, marjoram, sage, and tomatoes with their liquid. Mix well.

2. Cover tightly with foil. Bake 30 minutes. Uncover and stir in carrots, green beans, and parsley. Cover and bake 35 to 40 minutes longer, or until vegetables are tender. Remove bay leaves.

3. Sprinkle top with cheese and return to oven for a few minutes, until cheese melts.

199   SUPER CHEESE STRATA
Prep: 15 minutes   Cook: 45 minutes   Serves: 5 to 6

You can improvise on this basic dish. One time add leftover cooked chicken; another time add a few slivers of cooked ham, turkey, sausage, or bacon. You can also toss in a few canned drained corn kernels or some pimiento strips, if desired. Any way you make it, it's ideal brunch or supper fare.

2 tablespoons butter, at room temperature
6 slices white or sourdough bread, crusts removed
½ to ¾ pound mild cheddar cheese, shredded (2 to 3 cups)
3 eggs, beaten

2 cups milk
¼ teaspoon salt
1 teaspoon dry mustard, or 2 teaspoons prepared Dijon mustard
1 (4-ounce) can diced green chiles

1. Butter bread on both sides and cut into ½-inch cubes. Turn half of bread cubes and then half of cheese into a buttered 6 × 10-inch baking dish.

2. Add remaining bread cubes and remaining cheese.

3. Beat together eggs, milk, salt, mustard, and chiles until well blended. Pour over cheese and bread in dish. Cover and refrigerate overnight.

4. Preheat oven to 350°. Remove strata from refrigerator and uncover. Bake for 45 minutes, or until light and fluffy. Serve immediately.

NOTE: *To prepare strata in a 9 × 13-inch baking dish, use 10 slices bread, 1 pound cheese, 5 eggs, 3 cups milk, 1½ teaspoons dry mustard, and salt to taste. Makes 10 servings.*

200   CHILE CHEESE EGG BAKE
Prep: 10 minutes   Cook: 30 to 35 minutes   Serves: 8 to 10

Here's a version of the ever-popular quichelike dish that has been making the rounds for years. It's a winner. Serve as an entrée for brunch or dinner or as an appetizer, cut into small bite-size pieces.

10 eggs
½ cup flour
1 teaspoon baking powder
Dash of salt
1 (7-ounce) can diced green chiles

1 pint low-fat cottage cheese
1 pound Monterey Jack cheese, shredded

1. Preheat oven to 375°. In a large bowl, beat eggs with a wire whisk. Add flour, baking powder, and salt. Whisk until well blended.

2. Stir in chiles, cottage cheese, and Jack cheese; blend thoroughly. Turn into a greased 13x9x2-inch baking dish.

3. Bake 30 to 35 minutes, or until set in center. Cut into squares to serve.

201   SOUR CREAM CHEESY ENCHILADA CASSEROLE

Prep: 15 minutes   Cook: 30 to 35 minutes   Serves: 4 to 5

Delicious and easy to fix. Serve topped with sour cream, guacamole, shredded lettuce, and chopped tomatoes for a simple supper.

1 (10¾-ounce) can condensed creamy chicken mushroom soup
¾ cup sour cream
2 tablespoons milk
1 (4-ounce) can diced green chiles
2 scallions, chopped

9 (5¼-inch) corn tortillas
2 cups chopped cooked chicken
½ red bell pepper, chopped
½ pound cheddar cheese, shredded (2 cups)
1 (2.2-ounce) can sliced ripe olives, drained

1. Preheat oven to 350°. Mix together soup, sour cream, milk, chiles, and scallions.

2. Arrange 3 tortillas in bottom of an 11x7-inch baking dish. Sprinkle with half the chicken, then half the red pepper. Sprinkle with a third of the cheese, then top with a third of soup mixture, spreading evenly. Repeat layers. Top with remaining 3 tortillas, olives, remaining soup mixture, and then sprinkle with remaining cheese.

3. Bake 30 to 35 minutes, or until heated through and bubbly.

202   CHEESE QUICHE SUPREME

Prep: 15 minutes   Cook: 1¼ hours   Serves: 6

Wait until you taste this creamy quiche version made with cream cheese. It's one of my all-time favorite brunch offerings, with a vegetable salad and a goblet of cut-up fresh fruits.

1 sheet frozen puff pastry (half of a 17¼-ounce package)
1 (8-ounce) package cream cheese, cut into 8 equal pieces
6 eggs
1½ cups light cream or half-and-half
¼ teaspoon salt

¼ teaspoon pepper
1 tablespoon Dijon mustard
1 (4-ounce) can diced green chiles
3 cups shredded cheese (a combination of Gruyère or Swiss and white cheddar, or whatever else you like) (12 ounces)

1. Defrost puff pastry for 30 to 45 minutes. Preheat oven to 375°. On a lightly floured surface, roll out puff pastry to a circle 12½ inches in diameter. Fit without stretching into 10-inch quiche dish or deep-dish pie pan. Roll edges toward center of dish and press lightly against rim.

2. Place cream cheese pieces, spoke fashion, in bottom of crust. Beat together eggs, cream, salt, pepper, mustard, and chiles. Mix in cheese. Turn cheese filling into crust.

3. Place quiche on baking sheet (to catch any drips) and bake 1 hour and 15 minutes, or until a knife inserted in center comes out clean. Let cool for 5 minutes before cutting and serving.

NOTE: *Cubed cooked ham (1 cup) or crisp crumbled cooked bacon (½ cup) can be added to quiche along with cheese, if desired.*

203 MY FAVORITE QUICHE
Prep: 15 minutes   Cook: 35 to 40 minutes   Serves: 5 to 6

This is a dinner or brunch standby relied upon often at my house. Most often I prepare it without meat, but suit yourself. Ad lib and create different cheese and seasoning combinations, depending on what you have on hand. All you need to complete the meal is a tossed green or fresh fruit salad.

1½ **cups shredded cheddar cheese (6 ounces)**	7 **eggs**
1½ **cups shredded Monterey Jack cheese (6 ounces)**	⅓ **cup milk or light cream**
1 **cup chopped hickory-smoked cooked turkey breast or chopped baked ham (optional)**	¼ **teaspoon garlic salt**
	¼ **teaspoon pepper**
	1 **(4-ounce) can diced green chiles**
	¼ **cup chopped red bell pepper or pimiento**

1. Preheat oven to 375°. Sprinkle bottom of a buttered 9-inch round pie pan or shallow casserole with cheeses, then turkey.

2. In a medium bowl, whisk together eggs, milk, garlic salt, and pepper until thoroughly blended. Stir in green chiles and red pepper. Pour over turkey and cheeses.

3. Bake, uncovered, 35 to 40 minutes, or until set. Cut into wedges and serve immediately.

204   RAVIOLI BAKE

Prep: 10 minutes   Cook: 45 minutes   Serves: 6

No need to break apart and cook frozen ravioli prior to baking in this recipe. Simply layer sheets of the thawed ravioli in a baking dish with frozen broccoli and canned spaghetti sauce, then cover and bake. The results are delicious.

1 (27½-ounce) can spaghetti sauce with mushrooms
1 (17-ounce) package frozen cheese ravioli (50 ravioli), thawed

1 (16-ounce) package frozen cut broccoli spears, thawed
¼ cup grated Parmesan cheese

1. Preheat oven to 400°. Spoon 3 tablespoons spaghetti sauce evenly over bottom of an 11x7-inch (2-quart) rectangular baking dish.

2. Carefully fit half the ravioli sheets in a single layer on top of sauce in bottom of dish, breaking up only as necessary. (Do not separate ravioli into individual pieces). Top evenly with half the spaghetti sauce, then all of broccoli pieces. Place remaining ravioli, still in sheets, on top of broccoli. Top with remaining spaghetti sauce, spreading evenly. Sprinkle with cheese. Cover tightly with foil.

3. Bake 45 minutes, or until ravioli is tender and very hot in center. Let stand a few minutes before serving.

205   LASAGNE FLORENTINE

Prep: 20 minutes   Cook: 45 to 50 minutes   Serves: 6

There's no precooking of the noodles in this fuss-free lasagne. Simply assemble the dish and bake immediately. For speed, and ease, use a jar of store-bought spaghetti sauce, unless of course you have some homemade sauce handy in the freezer.

2 cups low-fat ricotta cheese
1 egg
¼ cup grated Parmesan cheese
¼ teaspoon garlic powder
1 (10-ounce) package frozen chopped spinach, thawed and squeezed dry

1 (32-ounce) jar spaghetti sauce with mushrooms, or 4 cups homemade spaghetti sauce
9 uncooked lasagne noodles
3 cups mozzarella cheese, shredded (¾ pound)

1. Preheat oven to 375°. In a medium bowl, combine ricotta cheese, egg, Parmesan cheese, garlic powder, and spinach. Mix to blend well.

2. Spread one third of spaghetti sauce over bottom of a 12x8-inch rectangular baking dish. Cover with 3 uncooked lasagne noodles. Top with half the ricotta cheese mixture and then sprinkle with 1 cup mozzarella cheese.

3. Spread with half the remaining spaghetti sauce. Top with another 3 noodles. Spread remaining ricotta cheese mixture over noodles and sprinkle with 1 cup mozzarella cheese.

4. Top with 3 remaining noodles, then spread on remaining spaghetti sauce. Sprinkle remaining 1 cup mozzarella cheese on top. Cover with foil.

5. Bake 45 to 50 minutes, or until noodles are tender. Let stand 5 minutes before serving.

206 SHORTCUT LASAGNE, MEXICAN STYLE
Prep: 15 minutes   Cook: 45 to 50 minutes   Serves: 6

Here's another fast lasagne that utilizes uncooked lasagne noodles. The flavoring here has Mexican overtones with the use of black beans and enchilada sauce. Cottage cheese and cheddar cheese are also included in this delicious and easy meatless dish.

1 **(10-ounce) can enchilada sauce**
1 **(14½-ounce) can cut-up, peeled tomatoes, undrained**
1 **(6-ounce) can tomato paste**
1 **(16-ounce) can black beans, rinsed and well drained**
9 **ounces lasagne noodles**
1 **pint (2 cups) low-fat cottage cheese**
3 **cups shredded cheddar cheese (¾ pound)**

1. Preheat oven to 375°. In a bowl, combine enchilada sauce, tomatoes with their juice, and tomato paste. Mix to blend well. Stir in black beans.

2. Spoon a third of tomato sauce mixture over bottom of a 12x8-inch rectangular baking dish. Top with 3 uncooked lasagne noodles. Spread evenly with 1 cup cottage cheese and sprinkle with 1 cup cheddar cheese. Spoon on half the remaining tomato sauce mixture.

3. Add another layer of 3 noodles, remaining 1 cup cottage cheese, then sprinkle with 1 cup cheddar cheese.

4. Add remaining 3 noodles in a single layer, remaining tomato sauce, and remaining 1 cup cheddar cheese. Cover tightly with foil.

5. Bake 45 to 50 minutes, or until noodles are tender. Let stand at least 5 minutes before serving.

207 SPINACH PIE

Prep: 15 minutes   Cook: 40 to 45 minutes   Serves: 6

This pie freezes well and makes wonderful brunch or picnic fare.

1 **(15-ounce) package all-ready pie crusts ***	1 **cup chopped scallions**
1½ **teaspoons flour**	1 **cup ricotta cheese**
2 **(10-ounce) packages frozen chopped spinach, thawed and squeezed dry**	5 **eggs**
	½ **cup grated Parmesan cheese**
	½ **pound baked ham, chopped**
	¼ **teaspoon pepper**

1. Preheat oven to 425°. Remove 1 pie crust from package and let stand at room temperature for 15 to 20 minutes. Unforld crust and peel off top plastic sheet. Press out fold lines and repair any cracks by pushing dough together with fingers (dampened, if necessary). Sprinkle flour over crust to edges. Place crust, floured side down, in a deep 9-inch glass pie dish. Peel off plastic sheet, easing crust into dish. Then press dough firmly against bottom and up sides of dish.

2. In a medium bowl, combine spinach, scallions, ricotta cheese, 4 eggs, and Parmesan cheese. Beat together to blend well. Stir in ham and pepper. Turn filling into pastry-lined dish.

3. Top with remaining crust. Cut top crust even with edge of pie dish. Reserve dough scraps. Fold edge of bottom crust over top crust, forming a rolled edge around dish. Flute edges of dough decoratively with fingers or fork tines. Cut a 1-inch hole in center of pie crust. Beat remaining egg and brush over top of pie.

4. Bake in center of oven for 20 minutes. Meanwhile, roll out reserved dough scraps and cut out flowers and leaves. After 20 minutes, remove pie from oven and arrange flowers and leaves over top (do not cover vent hole) of pie, using beaten egg to attach them. Brush tops of flowers and leaves with egg. Cover edges of pie with foil strips to prevent overbrowning.

5. Return pie to oven and continue baking 20 to 25 minutes, or until set. Let stand at least 15 minutes before serving.

* *Available in refrigerator section of supermarket.*

208 TUNA CHEESE PUFF
Prep: 10 minutes   Cook: 1 hour   Serves: 4 to 5

This recipe has been in my repertoire for years. It makes an appealing luncheon or supper dish and all you need to accompany it is a tossed green salad with a few assorted vegetables in it.

4 slices white bread, crusts removed
1 (6½-ounce) can tuna, drained, or ½ pound crab meat, rinsed and well drained
1½ cups shredded cheddar cheese (6 ounces)
1 (2-ounce) jar sliced pimientos, drained, or ¼ cup chopped red bell pepper

4 eggs
2⅔ cups milk
¼ teaspoon salt
⅛ teaspoon pepper
¼ teaspoon Worcestershire sauce
1½ teaspoons prepared yellow mustard

1. Preheat oven to 325°. Arrange bread in a single layer in bottom of greased 11 × 7-inch baking dish. Sprinkle evenly with tuna, ¾ cup cheese, and pimiento.

2. Beat together eggs, milk, salt, pepper, Worcestershire sauce, and mustard until well blended. Pour over tuna. Top with remaining ¾ cup cheese.

3. Bake 55 to 60 minutes, or until golden and puffed.

209 TUNA RICE CASSEROLE
Prep: 5 minutes   Cook: 40 minutes   Serves: 4

This recipe couldn't be simpler. Prepare a green salad while the casserole is in the oven and then relax.

1 cup long-grain white rice
1 (10¾-ounce) can condensed cream of mushroom soup
1¼ cups milk
1 (6½- or 7-ounce) can tuna packed in water, drained and flaked

¾ cup cottage cheese
3 scallions, chopped
¼ cup canned diced green chiles (optional)
1 cup frozen peas, thawed
1 cup crushed potato chips

1. Preheat oven to 400°. In a 2-quart casserole, combine rice, soup, milk, tuna, cottage cheese, scallions, and chiles. Blend until well mixed.

2. Cover dish with foil. Bake 25 minutes. Remove foil and stir in peas. Sprinkle crushed potato chips over top. Return to oven and continue baking 15 minutes longer, or until rice is tender.

210   SALMON AND POTATO SCALLOP
Prep: 10 minutes   Cook: 30 to 35 minutes   Serves: 4

This shortcut dish uses a packaged potato mix for the base instead of fresh potatoes.

1 (10-ounce) package frozen chopped spinach, thawed, excess moisture squeezed out
1 (5.25-ounce) package sour cream 'n' chive scalloped potato mix

1 (1-ounce) package ranch-style salad dressing mix
2 cups boiling water
1 cup milk
1 (6½-ounce) can pink salmon, drained

1. Preheat oven to 400°. In a 2-quart baking dish, layer half of each of the following: spinach, potatoes, seasoning from potato mix, and dry salad dressing mix. Pour on 1 cup boiling water and ½ cup milk. Top with all of salmon, distributing evenly.

2. Repeat layers with remaining ingredients in same order, ending with milk.

3. Cover with aluminum foil and bake 30 to 35 minutes, or until hot and bubbling. Let stand 5 minutes before serving.

211   OVERNIGHT SEAFOOD AND MACARONI CASSEROLE
Prep: 5 minutes   Cook: 1 hour   Serves: 4 to 5

This dish is a breeze to prepare ahead and refrigerate overnight. An hour before serving, bake in a preheated oven.

8 ounces imitation crab, rinsed several times and drained, or 1 (6½-ounce) can tuna packed in water, drained
1 (10¾-ounce) can condensed cream of celery or cream of mushroom soup
1 cup milk

1 cup small elbow macaroni or shell pasta
2 tablespoons minced fresh or freeze-dried chives
1 cup shredded cheddar or American cheese (4 ounces)
1 (10-ounce) package frozen peas and carrots, thawed

1. In a 1½-quart casserole dish with cover, combine all ingredients except peas and carrots; mix well. Cover dish and refrigerate 8 hours, or overnight.

2. Preheat oven to 350°. Bake, covered, 45 minutes. Stir in peas and carrots. Bake 10 to 15 minutes longer, or until set.

212   BAKED RED SNAPPER OLÉ
Prep: 10 minutes   Cook: 25 minutes   Serves: 4 to 6

This is a terrific way to prepare fish. It takes little effort, tastes good, and looks attractive. Tasters gave it high marks—a sure winner.

2 (10-ounce) packages frozen chopped spinach, thawed and squeezed dry
1 (4½-ounce) jar sliced mushrooms, rinsed and drained
3 scallions, chopped
1 (12-ounce) jar mild green chile salsa
1¼ to 1½ pounds fresh red snapper fillets
½ cup shredded Monterey Jack cheese (2 ounces)

1. Preheat oven to 425°. Line an 8 × 12-inch rectangular baking dish evenly with spinach. Sprinkle mushrooms and then scallions over spinach.

2. Pour half the salsa over all. Lay fish in single layer on top of salsa and vegetables. Top fish with remaining salsa.

3. Bake, uncovered, 20 to 25 minutes, or until fish is just opaque throughout. Sprinkle with cheese. Return to oven for 2 to 3 minutes, until cheese melts.

213   BAKED FISH IN MUSHROOM SAUCE
Prep: 5 minutes   Cook: 25 minutes   Serves: 4 to 5

This is a versatile dependable recipe for baked fish.

1 (15-ounce) can sliced potatoes, rinsed and drained
2 medium zucchini, shredded (2½ to 3 cups)
2 medium carrots, peeled and shredded
1 (10¾-ounce) can condensed cream of mushroom soup
¼ cup dry white wine
2 scallions, chopped
2 tablespoons chopped parsley
1 to 1½ pounds white fish fillets, such as sole, flounder, snapper, or cod
  Juice of 1 lemon
3 tablespoons grated Parmesan cheese

1. Preheat oven to 425°. Arrange potatoes, zucchini, and carrots evenly in bottom of a 12 × 8-inch rectangular baking dish.

2. Combine undiluted soup, wine, scallions, and parsley; mix until blended. Pour half of soup mixture over vegetables, spreading evenly with a rubber spatula. Arrange fish in a single layer over all; sprinkle with lemon juice. Pour remaining soup mixture over fish. Sprinkle cheese on top.

3. Bake about 25 minutes, or until fish is just opaque throughout. To serve, use a wide spatula to remove from dish.

214 CRAB PUFF
Prep: 5 minutes   Cook: 40 to 45 minutes   Serves: 4 to 5

This tasty offering goes together in minutes. Accompany with a green salad or fruit salad bowl.

½ **pound Monterey Jack cheese, sliced**
6 **eggs**
⅓ **cup milk**
½ **pound frozen snow crab, thawed, rinsed, and drained (or use imitation crab, if desired)**

1 **(4-ounce) can diced green chiles**
3 **scallions, chopped**
½ **teaspoon salt**
⅛ **teaspoon pepper**

1. Preheat oven to 350°. Line a greased 9-inch pie dish with cheese slices. Beat together eggs, milk, crab, chiles, scallions, salt, and pepper. Pour over cheese in pie dish.

2. Bake 40 to 45 minutes, or until just set in center. Cut into wedges.

215 BAKED STUFFED FRENCH TOAST
Prep: 15 minutes   Cook: 35 minutes   Serves: 4 to 5

Ideal for breakfast or brunch, this dish can be prepared the night before serving, if desired. Be sure to accompany with maple or assorted fruit syrups.

4 **large slices sourdough bread, crusts removed, bread cubed**
1 **(8-ounce) package cream cheese, cut into cubes**
1 **large Granny Smith apple, peeled and chopped**
6 **eggs**

1 **cup milk**
1½ **teaspoons ground cinnamon**
2 **to 3 tablespoons sifted powdered sugar**
   Maple syrup or apricot, blueberry, or raspberry syrup

1. Preheat oven to 375°. Place half the bread cubes in an ungreased 11 × 7-inch baking dish. Cover with all of cream cheese cubes, distributing evenly. Sprinkle with chopped apple. Top evenly with remaining bread cubes.

2. Beat together eggs, milk, and cinnamon until well blended. Pour over bread mixture in dish. Bake about 35 minutes, or until set. Sprinkle with powdered sugar. Serve with maple or a fruit syrup.

NOTE: *If desired, the prepared unbaked casserole can be covered with plastic wrap and refrigerated overnight. Follow directions above for baking temperature and time.*

Chapter 6

Slow Cookers

The electric slow cooker or crockery pot (known to most of us by its brand name—Crock-Pot®) is something I always felt I could live without. But as I began testing recipes for this book and talking to friends and acquaintances, I discovered that cooks throughout the country are using the pots in ever-increasing numbers. More than three million slow cookers were purchased in 1988 alone.

They are simple to use and require no tending. With only limited planning and advance preparation, cooks can put a meal on the table effortlessly, and often economically, because the pots are well suited to utilizing less expensive, less tender cuts of meat.

Busy people find slow cookers a boon because they can toss the makings for dinner into the pot in the morning, turn it on the low heat setting, leave the house for the day, and return home to a delicious ready-to-eat home-cooked creation.

If you've heard rumors about safety, be reassured. Food technologists told me that even the low-heat temperature setting is sufficient to raise the internal temperature of food to 160 degrees, the point at which bacterial growth is stopped, within four hours. Be aware, however, that you must start out with cold food products, not items that are warm or have been thawing on the counter overnight.

The crockery-cooker is designed for slow, moist-heat cooking. Be sure to cover the pot with the lid for heat retention. As the foods get hot, the steam produced rises and condenses into liquids on the lid and then returns to the food in the pot. Keep in mind that liquids don't boil away as in conventional cooking, so use the exact amount of liquid specified in the recipe.

You can estimate that recipes with uncooked vegetables and meats will take 8 to 10 hours on the low-heat setting. To speed cooking time, the high-heat setting can be used. Also, foods can be started on the high setting and then turned down. One hour on high is equal to about 2 to 2½ hours on low. The pots should never be used for reheating foods.

Slow cookers are available in a variety of sizes and designs and with an assortment of features. Some have removable casseroles or crocks that can be used on top of the stove or in the oven. The pots are available with plastic or glass lids and low and high temperature settings; some models have several heat choice settings. One brand even offers an Automatic Temperature Shift feature, which cooks the food on high heat the first 1¾ hours and then automatically shifts to low for the remaining cooking time.

When buying an electric slow cooker, suit your personal cooking style and needs. I found the 6-quart size the most versatile; the smaller sizes considerably limited the amount of foods that could be cooked.

After finding out how convenient the latest model crockery-cookers are, I'm convinced they belong in every home. I hope you find the recipes in this chapter as delicious as my unofficial family and friend tasting panel did.

216 CROCKERY POT OLD-FASHIONED VEGETABLE BEEF SOUP

Prep: 10 minutes   Cook: 8 to 9 hours   Serves: 4 to 5

Toss everything in the slow-cooking pot, turn the heat on the low setting, and in 8 hours you'll have a pot of soup to put on the table.

1 medium leek (white and tender green), washed well and chopped
3 celery ribs, chopped
6 carrots, peeled and chopped
1 (10.5-ounce) can corn kernels, drained
3 baking potatoes, peeled and cut into ½-inch cubes
1 pound boneless beef chuck or round steak, trimmed of all fat and cut into ½-inch cubes

1 (14½-ounce) can stewed tomatoes, undrained
¼ cup tomato paste
3 cups water
1 teaspoon salt
½ teaspoon pepper
2 garlic cloves, minced
1 individual serving-size packet powdered instant beef broth

1. In a 6-quart electric crockery-cooker, combine all ingredients. Stir to mix well.

2. Cover and cook on low-heat setting 8 to 9 hours, or until meat is tender.

217   BARBECUED BEEF AND BEANS
Prep: 15 minutes   Cook: 6½ to 7 hours   Serves: 5 to 6

Here's an easy way to fix barbecued beef and beans in a slow cooker.

1 (15¼-ounce) can kidney
   beans, rinsed and drained
1 (15-ounce) can pinto beans,
   rinsed and drained
1 (15-ounce) can Great
   Northern (large white)
   beans, rinsed and drained
2 medium green bell peppers,
   chopped

2 large onions, chopped
3 pounds boneless beef chuck
   roast, trimmed of all fat
   and cut into 1½-inch
   cubes
1½ cups bottled barbecue sauce
6 French rolls, halved

1. In a 6-quart electric crockery-cooker, combine kidney beans, pinto beans, Great Northern beans, green peppers, and onions. Top with beef cubes. Pour 1 cup barbecue sauce over all. Do not mix.

2. Cover and cook on high-heat setting 1 hour.

3. Reduce heat setting to low and cook, covered, 5 hours.

4. Remove cover and stir in remaining ½ cup barbecue sauce. Cook, uncovered, ½ to 1 hour longer. Serve over split French rolls.

218   SMOKY BEEF WITH BLACK-EYED PEAS
Prep: 15 minutes   Cook: 10 hours   Serves: 4

. The wonderful smoky flavor that permeates this dish comes from a can of bean with bacon soup. No substitutes, please!

1 (11½-ounce) can bean with
   bacon soup
1 (4-ounce) can diced green
   chiles
½ cup water
1 teaspoon garlic powder
1 teaspoon paprika
1 (9-ounce) package frozen
   black-eyed peas, slightly
   thawed

2 carrots, cut into ¼-inch-thick
   slices
1 medium onion, sliced
1½ pounds boneless beef chuck
   roast, trimmed of all fat
½ teaspoon salt

1. In a 4-quart electric crockery-cooker, combine undiluted soup, green chiles, water, garlic powder, paprika, black-eyed peas, carrots, and onion. Mix to blend well. Place roast down into mixture, covering top with some of it.

2. Cover and cook on low-heat setting for 10 hours. Stir in salt.

219 CROCKERY COOKER SOUPY-STYLE BEEF STEW

Prep: 15 minutes   Cook: 9 to 9½ hours   Serves: 6

This change-of-pace soupy-stew combines yams, green beans, orange juice, and cinnamon for some wonderfully appealing and satisfying eating.

2 medium onions, sliced
8 carrots, peeled and thinly sliced
3 sweet potatoes, peeled and sliced ½ inch thick
4 celery ribs, sliced
½ pound fresh green beans, cut into 1-inch pieces

3½ to 4 pounds boneless beef chuck roast, trimmed of all fat
¾ cup orange juice
¾ cup beef broth
½ teaspoon ground cinnamon
½ teaspoon salt
¼ teaspoon pepper

1. In a 6-quart electric crockery-cooker, layer onions, carrots, sweet potatoes, celery and green beans. Place roast on top.

2. In a medium bowl, mix together orange juice, broth, cinnamon, salt, and pepper. Pour over meat. Do not mix.

3. Cover and cook on high-heat setting 1½ hours.

4. Reduce heat setting to low and cook 7½ to 8 hours, until meat is very tender. Season with additional salt and pepper to taste.

220 POLISH SAUSAGE AND CABBAGE

Prep: 20 minutes   Cook: 7 to 8 hours   Serves: 6

Here's an easy way to make sausage and cabbage; no tending is required.

1½ pounds green cabbage, sliced or coarsely shredded
2 medium onions, chopped
3 medium russet potatoes, peeled and diced
1 red bell pepper, chopped
2 garlic cloves, minced
⅔ cup dry white wine

1½ pounds Polish kielbasa or smoked beef sausage, cut into 1-inch slices
1 (28-ounce) can cut-up, peeled tomatoes, undrained
1 tablespoon Dijon mustard
¾ teaspoon caraway seeds
½ teaspoon pepper

1. In a 6-quart electric crockery-cooker, combine cabbage, onions, potatoes, red pepper, garlic, wine, sausage, tomatoes with their liquid, mustard, caraway seeds, and pepper. Mix well.

2. Cover. Cook on low-heat setting 7 to 8 hours, or until cabbage is tender.

221   SLOW COOKER TEX-MEX STEAK AND RICE
Prep: 15 minutes   Cook: 5½ hours   Serves: 8

Be sure to use converted rice in this recipe because it holds its shape better in a slow cooker than other types of rice.

2 cups converted rice
2 medium onions, chopped
1 (7-ounce) can diced green chiles
3 celery ribs, chopped
1 medium green bell pepper, chopped
1 (1.25-ounce) package taco seasoning mix
1 (28-ounce) can cut-up, peeled tomatoes, undrained

1 (28-ounce) can crushed tomatoes with added puree
3 cups water
2 pounds boneless top round steak, trimmed of all fat and cut into 1-inch cubes
1 (10-ounce) package frozen French-style green beans

1. In a 6-quart electric crockery-cooker, combine rice, onions, chiles, celery, green pepper, taco mix, tomatoes with their liquid, and tomatoes with puree, water, and beef. Mix to blend well.

2. Cover and cook on high-heat setting 1½ hours.

3. Reduce heat setting to low and cook, covered, 4 hours, or until meat is tender. Last hour of cooking time, stir in green beans.

222   LAZY BEEF STEW
Prep: 20 minutes   Cook: 7 to 8 hours   Serves: 6 to 8

2 medium onions, chopped
4 celery ribs, chopped
5 russet potatoes, peeled and cut into ½-inch dice
6 carrots, peeled and cut into ¾-inch slices
1 green bell pepper, chopped
2½ pounds beef round steak, cut into 1½-inch cubes

1 (0.75-ounce) envelope mushroom gravy mix
½ cup dry white wine
1 (6-ounce) can tomato paste
½ teaspoon salt
½ teaspoon pepper
1 (16-ounce) package frozen French-style green beans, thawed

1. Turn a 6-quart electric crockery-cooker on high-heat setting while preparing ingredients. In crockery pot, mix together onions, celery, potatoes, carrots, green pepper, beef, dry gravy mix, wine, tomato paste, salt, and pepper.

2. Cover, reduce heat setting to low, and cook 7 to 8 hours, or until meat and vegetables are tender. Stir in green beans last ½ hour of cooking time.

223 VEAL ROAST WITH SHERRY-MUSTARD SAUCE
Prep: 20 minutes   Cook: 10 hours   Serves: 4 to 6

Be sure to purchase close to 3 pounds veal for this wonderfully seasoned creation made in a slow cooker. Depending on the size of the roasts available, you may need two.

2 (10¾-ounce) cans condensed golden mushroom soup
1 (4.5-ounce) jar sliced mushrooms, drained
1 tablespoon prepared yellow mustard
½ cup dry sherry
½ teaspoon ground turmeric
¼ teaspoon pepper
¾ pound carrots, quartered lengthwise and cut into 2-inch pieces

1½ pounds red potatoes, scrubbed and cut into 1-inch cubes
2¾ pounds boneless veal shoulder roast(s), trimmed of any excess fat
1 (16-ounce) package frozen French-style green beans, thawed

1. Turn a 5- or 6-quart electric crockery-cooker to high-heat setting while preparing ingredients. In cooker, mix together undiluted soup, drained mushrooms, mustard, sherry, turmeric, and pepper. Stir in carrots and potatoes. Nestle roast down in mixture and cover with some of sauce and vegetables.

2. Cover and reduce heat setting to low. Cook 9½ hours.

3. Place thawed green beans on top, cover, and cook 30 minutes longer.

224 EASY PORK CHILE VERDE
Prep: 20 minutes   Cook: 10 hours   Serves: 4 to 6

2 (7-ounce) cans green chile salsa
1 (7-ounce) can diced green chiles
1½ pounds boneless pork shoulder, cut into ½-inch cubes
1 pound fresh or canned (undrained) tomatillos (see Note)
9 garlic cloves, mashed
2 carrots, peeled and sliced ¼-inch thick

1 large russet potato, peeled and cut into ¼-inch cubes
1 large onion, halved and cut into ¼-inch slices
½ teaspoon salt
¼ teaspoon cayenne
2 medium tomatoes, chopped
½ cup chopped fresh cilantro or parsley
1 bunch scallions, thinly sliced
½ cup sour cream
1 dozen warm flour tortillas

1. Turn a 4- or 6-quart electric crockery-cooker on high-heat setting while preparing ingredients. Add salsa, chiles, pork, tomatillos, garlic, carrots, potato, and onion to cooker. Mix thoroughly.

2. Cover and reduce heat setting to low. Cook 10 hours without removing cover.

3. Stir in salt and cayenne. Serve with tomatoes, cilantro, scallions, sour cream, and warm tortillas, as accompaniment.

> **NOTE:** *If using fresh tomatillos, peel off papery skin and halve tomatillos.*

---

225   CHICKEN NEW ORLEANS
Prep: 20 minutes   Cook: 6 hours   Serves: 4

Béarnaise sauce mix lends interesting flavor to this simple and delicious dish.

2 (0.9-ounce) packages béarnaise sauce mix
½ cup dry white wine
½ teaspoon tarragon
½ teaspoon ground turmeric
½ teaspoon garlic powder
3 shallots, minced
1 pound cooked ham, cut into 1-inch chunks

1 red bell pepper, chopped
1 pound red potatoes, scrubbed and cut into ½-inch cubes
1 (9-ounce) package frozen artichoke halves and quarters, thawed
1 pound skinless chicken breast tenders

1. Turn a 4-quart electric crockery cooker on high-heat setting while preparing ingredients. In crockery pot, mix together both packages of béarnaise sauce mix, wine, tarragon, turmeric, and garlic powder until well blended. Add shallots, ham, red pepper, potatoes, artichokes, and chicken. Stir gently.

2. Cover, reduce heat setting to low, and cook 6 hours.

226   CHICKEN AND DUMPLINGS
Prep: 15 minutes   Cook: 6¼ hours   Serves: 6 to 8

2 medium onions, coarsely chopped
8 medium carrots, cut into ½-inch slices
4 celery ribs, chopped
3 cups frozen hash brown potatoes (about 1 pound), or chopped peeled baking potatoes
1 cup frozen corn kernels
1 (4-ounce) can mushroom stems and pieces, drained

1½ pounds skinless, boneless chicken breasts, cut into 1-inch chunks
2 (10¾-ounce) cans condensed golden mushroom soup
¼ cup dry white wine
½ teaspoon pepper
1 (16-ounce) package frozen peas, thawed
1 cup buttermilk baking mix, such as Bisquick
⅓ cup water

1. Turn a 6-quart electric crockery-cooker on high-heat setting while preparing ingredients. In crockery pot, combine onions, carrots, celery, potatoes, corn, mushrooms, chicken, undiluted soup, wine, and pepper. Mix well.

2. Cover, reduce heat setting to low, and cook 5½ hours.

3. Stir in peas. To make dumplings, mix together baking mix and water until well blended. Drop spoonfuls in 5 or 6 mounds on top of chicken mixture. Cover and cook ½ hour. Uncover and cook 15 minutes longer.

227   CHICKEN CHILI
Prep: 15 minutes   Cook: 5 to 6 hours   Serves: 8

This chili rendition is a breeze to put together with canned beans. Serve topped with shredded cheese, lettuce, and guacamole.

2 medium onions, chopped
1 red bell pepper, chopped
1 (7-ounce) can diced green chiles
1½ pounds skinless, boneless chicken breasts, cut into 1-inch chunks
2 teaspoons minced garlic
1 (28-ounce) can cut-up, peeled tomatoes, undrained

1 (12-ounce) can tomato paste
2 (16-ounce) cans black beans, rinsed and drained
2 (15-ounce) cans Great Northern (large white) beans, rinsed and drained
1 to 1½ tablespoons chili powder
¾ teaspoon oregano
½ teaspoon salt

1. Turn a 6-quart electric crockery-cooker on high-heat setting while preparing ingredients. In crockery pot, gently mix together onions, red pepper, chiles, chicken, garlic, tomatoes with their liquid, tomato paste, black beans, Great Northern beans, chili powder, oregano, and salt.

2. Cover. Reduce heat setting to low and cook 5 to 6 hours, or until chicken is cooked through and vegetables are tender.

Chapter 7

Pressure Cookers

When time is at a premium and the pressure is on to put a meal on the table fast, rely on the pressure cooker.

Unlike the relics of the past, today's pressure cookers are sleek and contemporary, with foolproof safety locks and valves and user-friendly features. It's no wonder they are making a comeback.

Pressure cookers not only cook foods quickly, evenly, and nutritiously (little oil is needed and fewer vitamins and minerals are lost), but yield homey-tasting comfort foods, such as one-dish soups, stews, and bean meals, that taste as though they've been simmering for hours. And the good news is that the dishes often take only a third or half the time required in conventional cooking. You get hours of flavor in short order.

Unlike the microwave oven, the amount of food in the pressure cooker doesn't affect the cooking time. It's the steam build-up in the sealed pressure cooker that creates pressure.

Pressure cookers are available in an array of sizes ranging from 4- to 9-quart. When purchasing, select the size to best suit your family's needs and lifestyle. And in case you're unsure about investing in this kitchen gadget, keep in mind that the pressure cooker is versatile and can double as a stockpot or steamer for conventional cooking.

Before using the pan, be sure to read the manufacturer's instruction manual thoroughly to understand how to lock the lid, regulate the heat, reduce pressure, and release the lid. It will also give you guidelines about foods suitable to cook in your particular model.

To get you in the swing of pressure cooking, start with any one of the hearty recipes that follow. Black Beans with Smoked Sausage, Smoky Pork, Pineapple, and Potato Stew, French-Style Cassoulet Stew, and Navy Bean Soup with Spicy Sausage are a few of the selections. Just wait until you taste them!

228   SMOKED OYSTER CHOWDER
Prep: 10 minutes   Cook: 45 to 50 minutes   Serves: 6

Canned oysters add a novel twist to this wonderfully satisfying chowder.

2½ pounds potatoes, peeled
     and cut into ½-inch cubes
     (about 6 cups)
1 large onion, chopped
2 (14½-ounce) cans chicken
     broth
3 cups water
1 cup light cream or half-and-
     half

1 (1-pound) package frozen
     mixed vegetables, thawed
2 (3¾-ounce) cans smoked
     oysters, drained and
     rinsed
¼ teaspoon salt
¼ teaspoon white pepper
½ cup chopped watercress or
     parsley

1. In a 6-quart pressure cooker, combine potatoes, onion, chicken broth, and water. Close lid and lock in place.

2. Place over high heat and bring to high pressure (about 15 minutes). Adjust heat to regulate and maintain high pressure and cook 10 minutes. Remove from heat and let pressure drop naturally, 15 to 20 minutes. Remove lid, tilting it away from you to allow any excess steam to escape.

3. Return pot to medium heat and add cream. With the back of a spoon or a potato masher, mash some of the potatoes. Add mixed vetetables, oysters, salt, and white pepper. Cook over medium heat just until vegetables and oysters are hot, about 5 minutes. Serve garnished with watercress.

229   LEEK AND POTATO SOUP WITH SHRIMP
Prep: 20 minutes   Cook: 35 minutes   Serves: 4 to 5

Using an electric hand mixer to puree the potato mixture and complete this soup in a single pot is a nifty trick.

3½ pounds russet potatoes,
     peeled and cut into 1-inch
     cubes
1 pound leeks (white and
     tender green), washed
     well and chopped
½ cup coarsely chopped celery
     tops
4 cups water

1 (14½-ounce) can chicken
     broth
1 teaspoon salt
½ teaspoon white pepper
1 pound frozen, shelled, and
     deveined large shrimp,
     rinsed and drained
1 cup heavy cream
¼ cup chopped parsley

1. In a 6-quart pressure cooker, combine potatoes, leeks, celery tops, and water. Close lid and lock in place.

2. Place over high heat and bring to high pressure (about 15 minutes). Adjust heat to regulate and maintain high pressure and cook 10 minutes. Reduce pressure with quick-release method by placing cooker in sink under cold running water. Remove lid, tilting it away from you to allow any excess steam to escape.

3. Using an electric hand beater, whip potato mixture for about 2 minutes, or until smooth. Discard any celery strings that collect on beater. Or puree in food processor or blender and return to pressure cooker. Mix in broth, salt, white pepper, shrimp, and cream. Cook, covered (no pressure), over medium heat, 10 minutes. Stir in parsley and serve.

---

230 HEARTY BEEF AND VEGETABLE SOUP WITH MUSHROOMS

Prep: 25 minutes   Cook: 45 minutes   Serves: 6

This from-scratch soup takes only three quarters of an hour in a pressure cooker.

1 large onion, chopped
2 carrots, peeled and sliced
3 garlic cloves, mashed
2 celery ribs, sliced
¼ cup chopped fresh cilantro
1½ pounds russet potatoes, peeled and cut into 1-inch chunks
2 pounds boneless beef chuck roast, trimmed of all fat and cut into 1½-inch cubes
1 (14½-ounce) can cut-up, peeled tomatoes, undrained

1 (14½-ounce) can beef broth
1 (12-ounce) bottle dark beer
½ pound Swiss chard or spinach, shredded
½ pound fresh mushrooms, sliced
2 teaspoons Worcestershire sauce
1 teaspoon salt
½ teaspoon pepper

1. In a 6-quart pressure cooker, mix together onion, carrots, garlic, celery, cilantro, potatoes, beef, tomatoes with their liquid, and broth. Close lid and lock in place.

2. Place over high heat and bring to high pressure (about 15 minutes). Adjust heat to regulate and maintain high pressure and cook 20 minutes. Reduce pressure with quick-release method by placing cooker in sink under cold running water. Remove lid, tilting it away from you to allow any excess steam to escape.

3. Stir in beer, Swiss chard, mushrooms, Worcestershire sauce, salt, and pepper. Return pot to stove and cook, covered (no pressure), over medium heat 10 minutes.

231   CHINESE SPARERIBS WITH BLACK BEAN SAUCE
Prep: 10 minutes   Cook: 40 minutes   Serves: 4

This dish is intriguing and rated top marks with tasters of all ages.

3 pounds country-style pork spareribs, cut into 3-inch chunks
½ cup Chinese black bean sauce
¼ cup dry sherry
¼ cup cider vinegar
1½ teaspoons Asian sesame oil
1 teaspoon ground ginger
½ teaspoon cayenne
1 (8-ounce) can sliced water chestnuts, drained

1 (6-ounce) package frozen Chinese pea pods
1 (16-ounce) package frozen pasta salad Orientale (a combination of Chinese noodles, broccoli, Chinese pea pods, water chestnuts, and red bell pepper)
6 scallions, chopped

1. Place rack in bottom of a 6-quart pressure cooker. Add spareribs. Mix together black bean sauce, sherry, vinegar, sesame oil, ginger, and cayenne; pour over spareribs. Close lid and lock in place.

2. Place over high heat and bring to high pressure (about 10 minutes). Adjust heat to regulate and maintain high pressure and cook 20 minutes. Reduce pressure with quick-release method by placing cooker in sink under cold running water. Remove lid, tilting it away from you to allow any excess steam to escape. Carefully remove hot rack.

3. Stir in water chestnuts, pea pods, pasta salad, and scallions. Mix well. Return pan to stove and cook, covered (no pressure), over medium-low heat 10 minutes.

232   SMOKY PORK, PINEAPPLE, AND POTATO STEW
Prep: 15 minutes   Cook: 35 to 40 minutes   Serves: 4 to 6

Liquid smoke is the secret to adding smoky flavor in this aromatic dish.

1 (20-ounce) can unsweetened pineapple chunks
2 pounds boneless pork shoulder, cut into 1½-inch cubes
2 carrots, peeled and sliced
1 medium green bell pepper, cut into 1-inch chunks
1 medium onion, chopped

1 teaspoon liquid smoke seasoning
2 tablespoons brown sugar
1 (24-ounce) package frozen potatoes O'Brien (with onions and peppers)
1 teaspoon salt
½ teaspoon pepper

1. Place rack in bottom of a 6-quart pressure cooker. Drain juice from pineapple into 1-cup measure. Add enough water to measure 1 cup; set aside.

2. Add pork cubes, carrots, green pepper, onion, liquid smoke, and reserved pineapple liquid to pressure cooker. Mix well. Do not add pineapple chunks. Close lid and lock in place.

3. Place over high heat and bring to high pressure (about 10 minutes). Adjust heat to regulate and maintain high pressure and cook 15 minutes.

4. Reduce pressure with quick-release method by placing cooker in sink under cold running water. Remove lid, tilting it away from you to allow any excess steam to escape. Carefully remove hot rack. Stir in brown sugar. Then gently stir in pineapple chunks, potatoes, salt, and pepper.

5. Return pot to stove and cook, covered (no pressure), over medium heat 10 to 15 minutes, until potatoes are tender.

233   FRENCH-STYLE CASSOULET STEW
Prep: 25 minutes   Cook: 1 hour 5 minutes   Serves: 4 to 6

This rendition of the involved French dish known as cassoulet takes just over an hour in the pressure cooker. And it tastes divine.

1 **(1-pound) package dried Great Northern beans, rinsed and picked over**
½ **pound frozen skinless chicken breast tenders, cut into 1-inch chunks**
½ **pound cooked ham, cut into 1-inch chunks**
½ **pound boneless lamb stew meat**
½ **pound hot smoked sausage links, cut into ½-inch-thick slices**
2 **tablespoons olive oil**
1 **large leek (white and tender green), washed well and cut into ½-inch pieces**

2 **carrots, peeled and sliced into ¼-inch rounds**
6 **garlic cloves, mashed**
2 **(14½-ounce) cans beef broth**
1½ **cups water**
½ **teaspoon ground cloves**
1 **teaspoon thyme**
1 **bay leaf**
½ **cup dry white wine**
1 **(14½-ounce) can cut-up, peeled tomatoes, undrained**
½ **teaspoon pepper**
¼ **teaspoon salt**
½ **cup chopped fresh parsley**

1. In a 6-quart pressure cooker, combine beans, chicken, ham, lamb, sausages, oil, leek, carrots, garlic, broth, water, cloves, thyme, and bay leaf. Mix well. Close lid and lock in place.

2. Place over high heat and bring to high pressure (about 10 minutes). Adjust heat to regulate and maintain high pressure and cook 40 minutes. Reduce pressure with quick-release method by placing cooker in sink under cold running water. Remove lid, tilting it away from you to allow any excess steam to escape.

3. Return pot to stove, place over medium heat, and add wine, tomatoes, pepper, and salt. Cook, uncovered, 15 minutes. Stir in parsley and serve.

234   NAVY BEAN SOUP WITH SPICY SAUSAGE
Prep: 15 minutes   Cook: 1 hour   Serves: 4 to 6

This tastes just like old-fashioned comfort food. Enjoy!

1 (1-pound) package dried
    Great Northern beans,
    rinsed and picked over
2 carrots, peeled and diced
2 celery ribs, chopped
1 green bell pepper, chopped
3 garlic cloves, minced
2 tablespoons olive oil
½ teaspoon thyme
½ teaspoon basil

1 bay leaf
¼ teaspoon cayenne
1½ quarts water
1 pound hot smoked sausage
    links, or any spicy garlic
    sausage, cut into ¼-inch
    slices
½ teaspoon salt
¼ cup chopped parsley

1. In a 6-quart pressure cooker, mix together beans, carrots, celery, green pepper, garlic, oil, thyme, basil, bay leaf, cayenne, and water. Close lid and lock in place.

2. Place over high heat and bring to high pressure (about 10 minutes). Adjust heat to regulate and maintain high pressure and cook 35 minutes. Reduce pressure with quick-release method by placing cooker in sink under cold running water. Remove lid, tilting it away from you to allow any excess steam to escape.

3. Stir in sausage and salt. Return pot to stove and cook, covered (no pressure), over medium-low heat 15 minutes. Stir in parsley and serve.

235   BLACK BEANS WITH SMOKED SAUSAGE
Prep: 15 minutes   Cook: 1 hour   Serves: 4 to 6

Cut cooking time for black beans in half by using a pressure cooker.

1 (1-pound) package dried
    black beans, rinsed and
    picked over
4 to 6 cups water
2 medium onions, coarsely
    chopped
7 garlic cloves, minced
2 tablespoons olive oil
3 celery ribs, sliced
3 small carrots, peeled and
    chopped
1 medium red bell pepper,
    chopped

Juice of 1 lemon
1 pound fully cooked Polish
    kielbasa sausage, cut into
    ¼-inch slices
1 teaspoon salt
¼ teaspoon pepper
¼ teaspoon cayenne
5 scallions, sliced
2 medium tomatoes, chopped
    Sour cream

1. In a 6-quart pressure cooker, combine beans, water (enough to cover) onions, garlic, oil, celery, carrots, and red pepper. Mix well. Close lid and lock in place. Place over high heat and bring to high pressure (10 to 15 min-

utes). Adjust heat to regulate and maintain high pressure and cook for 40 minutes.

2. Reduce pressure with quick-release method by placing cooker in sink and running cold water over it. Remove lid, tilting it away from you to allow any excess steam to escape.

3. Stir in lemon juice, sausage, salt, pepper, and cayenne. Return pot to stove and cook over low heat, stirring, until sausage is heated through, about 10 minutes. Serve in soup plates or bowls, garnished with scallions, tomatoes, and sour cream.

236   FIVE-BEAN TURKEY CHILI
Prep: 20 minutes   Cook: 1¼ hours   Serves: 4 to 6

Rely on the pressure cooker to speed up the preparation of the beans in this tasty dish. Do not attempt to leave out the 2 tablespoons oil. Oil must be used to control foaming of beans, which could clog the vent. Always clean the lid and vent well after cooking beans.

1 **medium green bell pepper, chopped**	1 **tablespoon chili powder**
1 **medium onion, chopped**	1½ **teaspoons ground cumin**
½ **cup dried red beans**	1½ **teaspoons oregano**
½ **cup dried pinto beans**	1 **teaspoon paprika**
½ **cup dried black-eyed peas**	½ **teaspoon cayenne**
½ **cup dried black beans**	1 **(15-ounce) can tomato sauce**
½ **cup dried pink beans**	2 **to 3 teaspoons salt**
9 **garlic cloves, mashed**	**Shredded cheddar cheese,**
1 **pound ground turkey**	**shredded lettuce, and**
2 **tablespoons olive oil**	**sour cream, as**
7 **cups water**	**accompaniment**

1. In a 6-quart pressure cooker, combine green pepper, onion, beans, garlic, turkey, oil, water, chili powder, cumin, oregano, paprika, and cayenne. Mix well. Close lid and lock in place.

2. Place over high heat and bring to high pressure (about 15 minutes). Adjust heat to maintain high pressure and cook 45 minutes. Reduce pressure with quick-release method by placing cooker in sink under cold running water. Remove lid, tilting it away from you to allow any excess steam to escape.

3. Stir in tomato sauce and salt. Return pan to stove and cook, uncovered, over medium heat 15 minutes. Serve in soup plates or bowls. Garnish with cheese, lettuce, and sour cream.

Chapter 8

Microwave

The microwave oven is a lifesaver for busy cooks on the go. It can help you turn out one-pot meals in a fraction of the time required in conventional cooking. And microwave cookery is cool, because the microwave doesn't heat up the kitchen the way a conventional stove or oven does.

With most of these easy-to-follow recipes, you'll be able to make dinner in 30 minutes or less from start to finish. All have been designed to cook and serve in the same dish. Muss and fuss are minimal as is cleanup. Just a single casserole or dish is all that is required.

In no time, you can whip up Easy Chop Suey, Microwave Vegetable Casserole, or Microwave Bean and Sausage Stew. Microwave Halibut and Vegetables is great for the fish brigade. Or when friends stop by unexpectedly and stay for dinner, whip up Microwave Southwest Chili to beat the clock. This unbeatable collection just scratches the surface of the microwave meal ideas that are possible.

Here are some basic tips for successfully microwaving one-pot meals. Use only microwave-safe glass and ceramic dishes. Keep in mind that casseroles can get hot, so use potholders when removing dishes from the oven. Use times in recipes as guidelines. Check dishes once or twice during cooking time, especially near the end, to avoid overcooking. Use round dishes for most even cooking and best results. Allow food to stand a couple of minutes to cool slightly before serving. And keep in mind that the recipes that follow have been designed for 600- to 700-watt ovens.

237   SHORTCUT GROUND BEEF STEW

Prep: 10 minutes   Cook: 25 minutes   Serves: 4 to 5

You'll be amazed at this quick stewlike concoction you can turn out from the microwave oven in less than half an hour. It's surprisingly delicious with ground beef. Even the teenager in my house approved wholeheartedly!

1 pound lean ground beef	1 (15-ounce) can sliced
1 medium onion, chopped	potatoes, drained
4 carrots, peeled and sliced	1 (4-ounce) can mushroom
2 garlic cloves, minced	stems and pieces, drained
1 (15-ounce) can tomato sauce	1 (9-ounce) package frozen
special (with tomato bits,	French-cut green beans
onions, celery, and green	2 teaspoons basil
peppers added)	¼ teaspoon pepper

1. In a 3-quart microwave-safe casserole with lid, combine ground beef and onion. Cook in microwave oven on High 3 minutes. Stir to break up lumps. Cook on High 4 minutes. Drain off fat.

2. Stir in carrots, garlic, and tomato sauce. Cover with lid. Cook on High 8 minutes.

3. Add potatoes, mushrooms, green beans, basil, and pepper. Cover and cook on High 10 minutes, stirring after 5 minutes.

238   MICROWAVE SOUTHWEST CHILI

Prep: 10 minutes   Cook: 30 to 35 minutes   Serves: 4 to 6

The microwave lends itself to making this terrific chili. Unsweetened chocolate and cinnamon add special flavor; don't omit them.

1 tablespoon vegetable oil	2 (16-ounce) cans black beans,
1 large onion, chopped	drained
1 garlic clove, minced	1 tablespoon chili powder
1 pound lean ground beef	¾ teaspoon ground cumin
1 (28-ounce) can cut-up,	½ teaspoon ground cinnamon
peeled tomatoes,	½ ounce (half of a 1-ounce
undrained	square) unsweetened
1 (6-ounce) can tomato paste	chocolate
1 (7-ounce) can diced green	
chiles	

1. In a 3-quart microwave-safe casserole, combine oil, onion, and garlic. Cook in microwave oven on High 4 minutes, stirring once.

2. Add beef and cook on High 4 minutes. Stir to break up lumps. Cook 3 to 4 minutes longer. Drain off any fat.

3. Stir in all remaining ingredients, mixing well. Cook on High, uncovered, 5 minutes. Stir. Cook 15 minutes longer, stirring once.

239 MICROWAVE SPAGHETTI WITH MEAT SAUCE AND GREEN BEANS
Prep: 10 minutes   Cook: 30 minutes   Serves: 6

This easy-on-the-cook microwave spaghetti dinner starts with uncooked spaghetti.

1 pound lean ground beef
1 onion, chopped
1 (28-ounce) jar spaghetti
   sauce
2 cups water
2 teaspoons basil

8 ounces thin spaghetti,
   broken into pieces
1 (9-ounce) package frozen
   Italian green beans
¼ cup grated Parmesan cheese

1. In a 3-quart microwave-safe casserole, combine beef and onion. Cook in microwave oven on High 4 minutes. Stir to break up any lumps. Cook on High 2 minutes longer. Drain off any fat.

2. Stir in spaghetti sauce, water, basil, and uncooked spaghetti; mix well.

3. Cover with lid and cook on High 5 minutes. Stir. Cover and cook on High 10 minutes longer. Stir in green beans. Sprinkle cheese over top. Cover and cook on High 7 to 8 minutes longer, or until spaghetti and green beans are tender.

240 HAMBURGER MACARONI SOUP
Prep: 5 minutes   Cook: 33 minutes   Serves: 4 to 5

This easy and delicious soup is a favorite with children and adults alike. Top with shredded cheese, if desired.

1 pound lean ground beef
1 medium onion, chopped
1 (28-ounce) can cut-up,
   peeled tomatoes,
   undrained
1 cup beef broth
2 cups water

1 cup elbow macaroni
2 teaspoons Worcestershire
   sauce
¾ teaspoon salt
¼ teaspoon pepper
1 (16-ounce) package frozen
   mixed vegetables

1. Crumble beef into a 5-quart microwave-safe casserole with lid. Add onion. In microwave oven, cook on High 6 minutes, stirring after 3 minutes to break up any lumps. Drain off fat. Cook on High 2 minutes longer. Drain off and discard any liquid.

2. Add tomatoes with their liquid, broth, water, macaroni, Worcestershire sauce, salt, and pepper. Cover with lid. Cook on High 15 minutes, stirring twice.

3. Add vegetables and stir well to break up. Cook, covered, on High 10 minutes, stirring once, until macaroni is tender.

241   TEX-MEX CHILI CORN SOUP
Prep: 10 minutes   Cook: 16 minutes   Serves: 4

When you're in the mood for a southwestern-style soup without much hassle, try this. It's terrific!

1 tablespoon butter
1 medium onion, chopped
1 (28-ounce) can cut-up, peeled tomatoes, undrained
1 (4-ounce) can diced green chiles
1 (11-ounce) can Mexicorn (whole kernel corn with red and green peppers), rinsed and drained

1 cup chicken broth
1 garlic clove, minced
1 cup shredded cooked chicken breast
1½ cups shredded Monterey Jack or cheddar cheese (6 ounces)

1. In a 3-quart microwave-safe casserole with lid, combine butter and onion. Cook in microwave oven on High 5 minutes, stirring once. Stir in tomatoes with their liquid, undrained green chiles, corn, broth, and garlic, mixing well. Cover with lid. Cook on High 10 minutes, stirring once, until soup comes to a full boil.

2. Stir in chicken. Cook, covered, on High 1 minute, until chicken is hot.

3. Stir in 1 cup cheese until well mixed. Serve immediately. Top each serving with a sprinkling of remaining ½ cup cheese.

242   TURKEY-STUFFED ACORN SQUASH WITH PINEAPPLE SAUCE
Prep: 10 minutes   Cook: 20 minutes   Serves: 4

Acorn squash makes a great container for a main dish as this recipe proves, and the microwave is the fastest way to cook it. Turkey, pineapple, and squash team together beautifully.

2 acorn squash, about 1 pound each
½ to ¾ pound ground turkey
½ onion, chopped
½ green bell pepper, chopped
2 carrots, peeled and shredded

1 tablespoon ketchup
¼ teaspoon salt
¼ teaspoon pepper
2 tablespoons converted rice
1 (20-ounce) can chunky pineapple sauce

1. Cut each squash in half lengthwise. Scoop out and discard seeds and stringy portion from center. Place squash, cut side up, in a shallow 2½-quart microwave-safe baking dish.

2. Combine turkey, onion, green pepper, carrots, ketchup, salt, pepper, and rice; mix well. Mound up and press into center of squash halves, dividing evenly. Top generously with pineapple sauce, using about half of it. Cover dish tightly with microwave-safe plastic wrap.

3. Cook in microwave oven on High about 15 minutes, rotating once. Remove from microwave and carefully remove plastic wrap. Top with remaining pineapple sauce; recover with plastic wrap. Return to microwave and cook on High 5 to 6 minutes longer, or until squash is very tender when pricked with a fork.

243 MICROWAVE SOUTHWEST CHICKEN
Prep: 10 minutes   Cook: 25 minutes   Serves: 4 to 5

This chicken is quick, attractive, and delicious. While the chicken stands after cooking, microwave the zippy vegetables. Add cayenne for a little heat, if desired.

1 (3½-pound) chicken, skin removed	2 medium zucchini, chopped (about 3 cups)
1½ teaspoons ground cumin	2 cups frozen corn kernels
1½ teaspoons chili powder	3 tomatoes, seeded and chopped
½ teaspoon paprika	
2 tablespoons red wine vinegar	

1. Remove giblets and neck from chicken and discard. Rinse chicken with cold water and pat dry with paper towels. Combine 1 teaspoon cumin, 1 teaspoon chili powder, paprika, and 1 tablespoon vinegar; mix well to make a paste. Rub all over outside of chicken. Place chicken, breast side down, in a deep 3-quart microwave-safe casserole. Cover with wax paper.

2. Cook in microwave on High for 9 minutes. Turn chicken breast side up, cover, and cook on High 9 to 12 minutes longer, or until juices run clear.

3. Place chicken on a serving platter. Skim off fat from drippings in casserole dish; then drain off all but ¼ cup drippings.

4. Add zucchini, corn, and tomatoes to drippings remaining in dish. Stir in remaining ½ teaspoon cumin, ½ teaspoon chili powder, and 1 tablespoon vinegar; mix well. Cover with wax paper. Cook on High 6 minutes, turning dish once, until vegetables are crisp-tender. Serve vegetables with chicken.

244   EASY CHOP SUEY
Prep: 5 minutes   Cook: 14 to 16 minutes   Serves: 4

If you have a yen for chop suey, make this American innovation in the microwave oven. Serve with hot cooked rice.

1 pound lean ground beef or turkey	1 (4-ounce) can mushroom stems and pieces, drained
6 scallions, chopped	1 (6-ounce) package Chinese pea pods, thawed
2 celery ribs, chopped	4 cups fresh bean sprouts (about 1 pound)
½ teaspoon garlic powder	
¼ teaspoon pepper	
3 tablespoons soy sauce	

1. Crumble beef into a 3-quart microwave-safe casserole with lid. Add scallions and celery. Cook in microwave oven on High 4 minutes. Stir to break up lumps. Drain off fat. Cook on High 3 to 4 minutes longer. Drain off fat.

2. Stir in garlic powder, pepper, soy sauce, mushrooms, pea pods, and bean sprouts.

3. Cover with lid. Cook on High 7 to 8 minutes, stirring once, until pea pods are crisp-tender and mixture is very hot.

245   CHICKEN NOODLE CASSEROLE
Prep: 10 minutes   Cook: 16 to 17 minutes   Serves: 4 to 5

A dinner-in-a-jiffy idea to serve from the microwave.

8 ounces medium egg noodles	½ cup coarsely chopped pimiento-stuffed green olives
1 cup water	
1 cup milk or chicken broth	½ teaspoon garlic powder
½ cup dry white wine	½ teaspoon salt
1 (16-ounce) package frozen broccoli, cauliflower, and red peppers	¼ teaspoon pepper
2 cups chopped cooked chicken	1 cup shredded cheddar cheese (4 ounces)

1. Combine noodles, water, and milk in a 3-quart microwave-safe casserole with a lid. Cover with lid and cook in microwave oven on High 6 minutes, stirring once.

2. Add wine, vegetables, chicken, olives, garlic powder, salt, and pepper. Cook, covered, on High 7 to 8 minutes, stirring once, until vegetables and noodles are tender.

3. Stir in ½ cup cheese. Sprinkle top with remaining ½ cup cheese. Cook on High 3 minutes, or until hot in center and cheese is melted.

246 SWEET-SOUR RED CABBAGE AND SAUSAGE
Prep: 10 minutes   Cook: 22 minutes   Serves: 4 to 5

Save cooking time by preparing red cabbage in the microwave oven. This dish reminds me of my grandmother's red cabbage, which was prepared without the sausage and, of course, required a considerably longer cooking time on top of the stove.

¾ **pound fully cooked Polish kielbasa sausage, cut into ¼-inch slices**
1 **medium head red cabbage, shredded (about 7 cups)**
2 **small tart green apples, chopped**

1 **medium onion, chopped**
3 **tablespoons red wine vinegar or cider vinegar**
3 **tablespoons water**
3 **tablespoons brown sugar**
½ **teaspoon salt**

1. In a 3-quart microwave-safe casserole with lid, cook sausage in microwave on High 5 minutes, stirring once. Drain off any fat. Remove sausage to a plate and set aside.

2. Add cabbage to same casserole along with apples, onion, vinegar, water, brown sugar, and salt. Cover casserole with lid and cook on High 10 minutes. Stir. Cook on High 5 minutes, or until cabbage is tender.

3. Stir in sausage and cook, covered, on High 2 minutes, until sausage is hot. Let stand, covered, 5 minutes before serving.

247 MICROWAVE BEAN AND SAUSAGE STEW
Prep: 10 minutes   Cook: 17 to 18 minutes   Serves: 4 to 5

With this dish, you can capture the flavor of bean stew in short order. Vary the canned beans according to your liking.

1 **medium onion, chopped**
3 **carrots, peeled and chopped**
1 **pound smoked beef sausage, sliced**
¼ **teaspoon thyme**
¼ **teaspoon rosemary, crushed**
2 **medium zucchini, chopped**
1 **(17-ounce) can green lima beans, rinsed and drained**

1 **(15-ounce) can cannellini (white kidney) beans or red kidney beans, rinsed and drained**
1 **(6-ounce) can tomato paste**
½ **cup dry white wine**
½ **teaspoon salt**
¼ **teaspoon pepper**

1. In a 3-quart microwave-safe casserole with lid, combine onion, carrots, sausage, thyme, and rosemary. Cover with lid. In microwave oven, cook on High 4 minutes. Drain off fat and liquid and discard.

2. Stir in zucchini, beans, tomato paste, wine, salt, and pepper; mix well. Cover. Cook on High 13 to 14 minutes, stirring twice, or until vegetables are tender.

248   BLACK BEAN SOUP WITH SHRIMP
Prep: 10 minutes   Cook: 30 minutes   Serves: 4 to 6

This quick variation on the black bean soup theme is made in the microwave oven. Since the beans haven't been cooked from scratch or pureed, don't expect a dark-looking broth.

1 medium onion, chopped	2 (16-ounce) cans black beans,
2 celery ribs, chopped	rinsed and drained
1 medium green bell pepper,	3 tablespoons dry sherry
chopped	1½ teaspoons ground cumin
2 carrots, peeled and chopped	½ pound frozen, shelled, and
2 garlic cloves, minced	deveined precooked
2 (14½-ounce) cans beef broth	medium shrimp, thawed
1 (14½-ounce) can cut-up,	1 tablespoon white wine
peeled tomatoes,	vinegar
undrained	¾ cup sour cream
1 cup water	

1. In a 5-quart microwave-safe casserole with lid, combine onion, celery, green pepper, carrots, garlic, broth, tomatoes with their liquid, and 1 cup water. Cover with lid and cook in microwave oven on High 18 minutes.

2. Stir in black beans, sherry, and cumin. Cover and cook on High 12 minutes.

3. Meanwhile rinse shrimp with cold water, drain, and sprinkle with vinegar.

4. To serve, ladle soup over several shrimp in soup bowls. Top each serving with a dollop of sour cream

249   TUNA RICE CASSEROLE
Prep: 10 minutes   Cook: 13 to 14 minutes   Serves: 4

The microwave oven comes to the rescue with this jiffy meal with tuna and rice. For best-tasting results, be sure to use the newer fast-cooking long-grain rice rather than the original precooked instant rice.

1½ cups fast-cooking long-grain	2 celery ribs, chopped
rice	½ cup chopped red bell pepper
1 (10¾-ounce) can condensed	1 (16-ounce) package frozen
cream of mushroom soup	French-style green beans
1 cup water	or peas
1 (6½-ounce) can tuna,	2 tablespoons dry white wine
drained and flaked	½ teaspoon salt
4 scallions, chopped	¼ teaspoon pepper

1. In a 3-quart microwave-safe casserole with lid, mix together all ingredients until well blended.

2. Cover with lid. Cook in microwave oven on High 13 to 14 minutes, stirring once, until beans are tender. Let stand, covered, 5 minutes before serving.

---

250   MICROWAVE HALIBUT AND VEGETABLES
Prep: 5 minutes   Cook: 14 to 16 minutes   Serves: 4

This is one of the fastest and most delicious ways to prepare fish. The recipe works well with soft as well as firm fish. Figure about 7 minutes of microwaving time per pound of fish.

1   (16-ounce) package frozen zucchini, mushrooms, pearl onions, and carrots, or any other frozen vegetable combination desired
1   pound halibut steaks, ¾ inch thick

1   lemon
1½ teaspoons dried dill weed
2   medium tomatoes, chopped
1   medium green bell pepper, chopped
¼   teaspoon garlic salt
⅛   teaspoon pepper

1. Place package of frozen vegetables on a double thickness of paper plates. Pierce holes with a knife in a couple of places in top of package. Cook in microwave on High 7 to 8 minutes, or until thawed and partially cooked. Drain off excess water; set vegetables aside.

2. Arrange fish in a 10-inch pie plate or oval microwave-safe baking dish. Squeeze juice of ½ lemon over fish and sprinkle with dill weed. Cover with microwave-safe plastic wrap. Cook in microwave on High 3½ minutes, turning dish once during cooking time. Remove from oven and drain off and discard any excess liquid from dish.

3. Place tomatoes, green pepper, and partially cooked vegetables on top and around sides of fish. Sprinkle with garlic salt and pepper. Squeeze juice of remaining ½ lemon over top. Cover with plastic wrap. Return to microwave and cook on High 3½ to 4½ minutes, or until fish flakes easily when pierced with a fork.

4. Serve fish with vegetables. Garnish with lemon wedges.

251   MICROWAVE VEGETABLE–COTTAGE CHEESE BAKE

Prep: 10 minutes   Cook: 18 to 20 minutes   Serves: 4 to 5

This main dish loaded with vegetables cooks in short order in the microwave oven. For a meatless dish, omit the chicken; it will serve 3.

1 (10-ounce) package frozen chopped spinach	2 eggs
1 (16-ounce) package frozen cut broccoli spears	1 cup cottage cheese
3 scallions, chopped	½ teaspoon salt
1 (12-ounce) can corn kernels, drained	¼ teaspoon pepper
2 cups diced cooked chicken or ham	1 teaspoon Worcestershire sauce
	1 cup shredded cheddar cheese (4 ounces)

1. Place spinach package in a 10-inch microwave-safe glass pie plate. In a microwave oven, cook on High 3 or 4 minutes, or until thawed. Drain spinach thoroughly, squeezing out as much moisture as possible.

2. Wipe out dish. In same dish, combine broccoli, scallions, and spinach. Cover with microwave-safe plastic wrap, leaving one end open to vent. Cook on High 6 to 7 minutes, until almost tender. Drain off all liquid, squeezing out as much as possible. Mix in corn and chicken.

3. In a small bowl, beat together eggs, cottage cheese, salt, pepper, and Worcestershire sauce. Pour over vegetable mixture. Cover with plastic wrap. Cook on High 7 minutes. Top with cheddar cheese, and cook uncovered on High 2 minutes, until cheese melts and eggs are set.

252   MICROWAVE VEGETABLE CASSEROLE

Prep: 15 minutes   Cook: 20 minutes   Serves: 4 to 5

Here's a simple meatless entrée selection for microwave devotees.

4 medium baking potatoes, peeled and thinly sliced	2 medium zucchini, sliced
1 bunch broccoli, trimmed and cut into 1-inch pieces (about 4 cups)	1 (10¾-ounce) can condensed cream of mushroom soup
1 medium onion, chopped	¼ cup dry white wine
3 large carrots, peeled and thinly sliced	¼ teaspoon garlic salt
	¼ teaspoon pepper
	1 cup shredded cheddar cheese (4 ounces)

1. In a shallow oval 2½-quart microwave-safe casserole, layer ingredients as follows: potatoes, broccoli, onion, and carrots. Cover with microwave-safe plastic wrap. In microwave oven, cook on High 10 minutes.

2. Add zucchini in an even layer. Cover and cook on High 2 minutes.

3. In a medium bowl, mix together undiluted soup, wine, garlic salt, pepper, and ½ cup cheese. Spoon over vegetables, spreading evenly. Cover with plastic wrap. Cook on High 4 minutes. Uncover and cook on High 3 to 4 minutes, or until potatoes are tender. Sprinkle with remaining ½ cup cheese and cook on High 1 minute, or until cheese is melted.

253 MICROWAVE SPAGHETTI SQUASH SUPREME

Prep: 10 minutes   Cook: 21 to 25 minutes   Serves: 4

Spaghetti squash is most easily prepared in a microwave oven. You save lots of time and energy. This version is meatless, but leftover cooked meat or poultry, such as ham, beef, chicken, or turkey, could easily be added to the sauce mixture.

1 **(3-pound) spaghetti squash**	¼ **cup chopped fresh basil**
2 **large tomatoes, chopped**	1 **tablespoon balsamic vinegar**
(about 2 cups)	2 **tablespoons drained capers**
1 **medium zucchini, chopped**	¾ **teaspoon salt**
3 **scallions, chopped**	¼ **teaspoon pepper**

1. With a large sharp knife or meat fork, pierce through skin of squash in several places (it will be tough). Place on a paper plate in microwave oven. Cook on High 8 minutes. Turn and cook on High another 8 to 12 minutes, or until skin of squash is tender and can be pierced easily. Set aside while making sauce.

2. In a 2-quart microwave-safe casserole, combine tomatoes, zucchini, and scallions. Cover with wax paper and cook on High 5 minutes, stirring once, until vegetables are crisp-tender. Stir in basil, vinegar, capers, salt, and pepper.

3. Cut squash in half and remove seeds. Using a fork or large serving spoon, remove squash strands from shell to serving platter. Top with vegetable sauce.

Chapter 9

Wok/Stir-Fry

When you fire up a wok and master the simple technique of stir-frying, you can deliver fabulous meals to the table in a flash. This quick-cooking method can be used for all kinds of good-looking and good-tasting recipes, from Chinese-inspired creations to innovative Western dishes. Use a wok to turn out Stir-Fry Chicken Fajitas, Chicken with Pineapple Salsa, Nectarine Chicken Curry, Chicken and Vegetable Pesto Stir-Fry, or Stir-Fried Chicken with Tomatillos and Papaya. Of course, if more traditional tastes appeal to you, try Kung Pao Shrimp, Sweet-and-Sour Walnut Chicken, Tomato Beef, Szechuan Shredded Chicken, or Orange Beef.

Since all the ingredients are cooked so quickly, it's essential that they be cut up and set out before you start cooking. Often the preparation time is more time-consuming than the actual cooking. But in many instances, foods can be chopped or cut up ahead and stored in plastic bags in the refrigerator.

To give recipes Oriental flavor and flair, invest in a few basics, such as Asian sesame oil, chili paste with garlic, hoisin sauce, and soy sauce. Found at Asian markets and in many supermarkets, these ingredients have a long shelf-life, and they can be mail-ordered if they are not available in your area.

When it comes to choosing a wok, get the best, heaviest one you can afford. My favorite is referred to as a Peking Pan. It's black, 12 inches in diameter, has sloping sides, and can be used for a variety of stove-top cooking. Season as instructed by heating or rubbing with a little vegetable oil.

254 STIR-FRIED BEEF AND PEPPERS
Prep: 15 minutes   Cook: 10 to 12 minutes   Serves: 4

This recipe allows you to get dinner on the table fast, once the chopping chores have been completed. To expedite the cooking, cut the meat and peppers the night before, wrap them separately, and refrigerate. Serve over plenty of hot cooked rice.

¼ cup beef broth
2 tablespoons reduced-sodium soy sauce
2 tablespoons dry sherry
1 teaspoon cornstarch
1 garlic clove, minced
¼ teaspoon pepper
1 pound boneless sirloin steak

3 tablespoons vegetable oil
1 medium red bell pepper, cut into thin strips
1 medium green bell pepper, cut into thin strips
1 (6-ounce) package frozen Chinese pea pods with water chestnuts, thawed

1. In a small bowl, combine beef broth, soy sauce, sherry, cornstarch, garlic, and pepper. Stir to dissolve cornstarch. Set sauce aside.

2. Trim any excess fat from steak. Cut beef into thin strips diagonally across the grain. In a wok or large skillet, heat 1 tablespoon oil. Add half the beef and stir-fry over high heat 2 to 3 minutes, until browned on outside but still pink inside. Remove to a plate. Repeat with another tablespoon oil and remaining beef; remove to plate with beef.

3. Add remaining 1 tablespoon oil to wok and heat until hot. Add red and green peppers and pea pods and stir-fry until crisp-tender, 3 to 4 minutes.

4. Reduce heat to medium-high. Stir sauce and add to wok. Stir-fry until sauce boils and thickens. Return beef to pan and cook until heated through, about 1 minute; do not overcook beef.

255 TOMATO BEEF
Prep: 15 minutes   Cook: 15 minutes   Serves: 6

This easy stir-fry is a longtime family favorite that you can whip together without much difficulty for a weeknight meal. Serve over hot rice.

1½ pounds boneless top sirloin or flank steak
3 tablespoons vegetable oil
1 large onion, cut into thin wedges
2 cups diagonally sliced celery
1 medium green bell pepper, cut into 1-inch chunks
1 teaspoon garlic salt
½ teaspoon ground ginger

2 tablespoons soy sauce
¼ cup beef broth
2 tablespoons ketchup
1 tablespoon red wine vinegar
1 tablespoon cornstarch
3 firm, ripe medium tomatoes, cut into eighths
1 (8-ounce) can sliced water chestnuts, drained

1. With a sharp knife, cut beef diagonally across the grain into thin strips. In a wok, heat 1 tablespoon oil over high heat until hot. Add half the beef and stir-fry quickly until meat loses its red color, about 3 minutes. Remove meat to a plate. Repeat with another tablespoon oil and remaining beef. Remove to plate.

2. Heat remaining 1 tablespoon oil over medium-high heat until hot. Add onion and celery and stir-fry 3 to 5 minutes, or until tender. Add green pepper and stir-fry 2 minutes, or until crisp-tender.

3. In a small bowl, mix together garlic salt, ginger, soy sauce, broth, ketchup, vinegar, and cornstarch. Add to wok along with tomatoes and water chestnuts. Mix well. Return beef to wok. Cook, stirring gently, over medium-high heat, 3 or 4 minutes, until sauce boils and thickens.

256   ORANGE BEEF
Prep: 20 minutes   Cook: 8 to 12 minutes   Serves: 4

This is a fragrant rendition of that popular Chinese favorite. It's delicious served over hot cooked rice.

1 **pound boneless top sirloin steak, partially frozen**	½ **to 1 teaspoon Chinese chili paste with garlic**
3 **tablespoons soy sauce**	2 **tablespoons frozen orange juice concentrate**
¼ **cup plus 1 teaspoon sugar**	1 **tablespoon ketchup**
1 **egg white**	¼ **cup plus 1 tablespoon water**
2 **tablespoons cornstarch**	**Few drops of orange extract (optional)**
2 **tablespoons vegetable oil**	**Minced fresh parsley and orange slices, for garnish**
2 **tablespoons finely chopped fresh orange or tangerine peel**	

1. Cut partially frozen steak across grain into paper-thin slices about 1½ inches long and 1-inch wide. In a medium bowl, combine 1 tablespoon soy sauce and 1 teaspoon sugar. Add beef slices and toss to coat. Marinate 5 minutes. Mix in egg white; then add 1 tablespoon cornstarch, mixing with fingers to distribute evenly.

2. In a wok or 10-inch skillet, heat oil over high heat until hot. Add beef and stir-fry until meat just loses its redness, about 3 minutes. With a slotted spoon, remove to a dish.

3. In oil remaining in wok, stir-fry orange peel over medium heat 2 to 3 minutes to soften. Mix in chili paste with garlic, orange juice concentrate, remaining 2 tablespoons soy sauce, remaining ¼ cup sugar, ketchup, ¼ cup water, and orange extract. Heat to boiling. Dissolve remaining 1 tablespoon cornstarch in remaining 1 tablespoon cold water and add to wok. Cook, stirring constantly, until sauce boils and thickens, 1 to 2 minutes.

4. Return beef to wok and heat through, 1 to 2 minutes. Garnish with minced fresh parsley and orange slices, if desired.

257 STIR-FRIED FLANK STEAK AND VEGETABLES

Prep: 10 minutes   Cook: 11 to 13 minutes   Serves: 4 to 5

A delicious quick dish, attractive enough to serve to guests. Accompany with pasta or rice and a mixed green salad.

2 tablespoons vegetable oil	¼ pound fresh mushrooms, sliced
1 pound flank steak, sliced across grain diagonally into thin strips	2 teaspoons minced garlic
2 scallions, chopped	¼ cup dry white wine
1 cup diced canned artichoke hearts	½ teaspoon black pepper
1 medium zucchini, cut into thin strips	1 (7-ounce) jar roasted red peppers, rinsed, drained, and cut into thin strips

1. In a wok or 10-inch skillet, heat 1 tablespoon oil over high heat. Add half the beef and stir-fry until browned outside but still rare inside, 2 to 3 minutes. Remove to a plate and set aside. Repeat with remaining oil and beef.

2. Add scallions, artichoke hearts, zucchini, mushrooms, and garlic to wok. Stir-fry 2 to 3 minutes, until crisp-tender.

3. Stir in wine, black pepper, and roasted red peppers. Toss over high heat until very hot, 1 to 2 minutes. Return beef to skillet and stir mixture together. Reduce heat to medium-low and cook until heated through, about 2 minutes.

258 BEAN CURD WITH MEAT SAUCE

Prep: 10 minutes   Cook: 10 minutes   Serves: 5 to 6

This is an adaptation of a recipe sampled in a cooking class in Hong Kong a few years ago. You won't recognize the tofu, as it takes on the flavors of the other ingredients in the dish.

1 pound firm bean curd (tofu)	½ teaspoon sugar
¼ teaspoon salt	3 teaspoons cornstarch
4 tablespoons vegetable oil	½ teaspoon Asian sesame oil
1 garlic clove, minced	⅛ teaspoon pepper
1 tablespoon minced fresh ginger	¼ cup chicken broth
2 scallions, finely chopped	2 tablespoons chopped mild or hot green chile pepper
1¼ teaspoons soy sauce	¾ cup frozen peas, thawed
½ pound lean boneless pork, finely chopped	

1. Cut tofu into small cubes and season with ⅛ teaspoon salt. In a wok, heat 2 tablespoons oil with garlic and ginger over medium heat until hot. Add scallions, tofu, remaining ⅛ teaspoon salt, and ¼ teaspoon soy sauce. Stir-fry 3 minutes and remove to a plate.

2. In a medium bowl, mix pork with remaining 1 teaspoon soy sauce, sugar, 1½ teaspoons cornstarch, ¼ teaspoon sesame oil, and pepper.

3. Heat remaining 2 tablespoons oil in same wok over high heat until hot. Add pork mixture and stir-fry 3 to 4 minutes, or until cooked through.

4. Dissolve remaining 1½ teaspoons cornstarch in broth and add to wok. Add chile pepper and remaining ¼ teaspoon sesame oil. Return bean curd to wok and stir in peas. Heat through, 2 to 3 minutes. Serve immediately.

259   STEAK SUEY
Prep: 15 minutes   Cook: 8 to 10 minutes   Serves: 4 to 5

This is an easy and tasty dish to whip up in a wok to stretch a half a pound of beef to serve 4 or 5. Serve over hot cooked rice or cooked Chinese water noodles. Or top with crispy chow mein noodles instead.

½ **pound boneless top sirloin steak**
2 **tablespoons vegetable oil**
3 **celery ribs, coarsely chopped**
4 **scallions, sliced**
3 **cups shredded green cabbage**
1 **(6-ounce) jar sliced mushrooms, rinsed and drained**

2 **cups fresh bean sprouts or 1 (16-ounce) can bean sprouts, rinsed and drained**
3 **tablespoons soy sauce**
1 **tablespoon dry sherry**
1 **tablespoon cornstarch**
¼ **cup beef broth**
¼ **teaspoon pepper**

1. Cut beef diagonally across grain into thin strips. Cut strips into slivers.

2. In a wok or large skillet, heat 1 tablespoon oil until very hot. Add beef and stir-fry over high heat until beef just loses its redness, about 2 minutes. Remove beef to a plate.

3. Heat remaining 1 tablespoon oil in wok until hot. Add celery, scallions, and cabbage. Stir-fry over high heat until cabbage is tender, 3 to 4 minutes. Add mushrooms, bean sprouts, soy sauce, and sherry. Cook, tossing, until heated through, 1 to 2 minutes.

4. Blend cornstarch with beef broth, stirring to dissolve. Add to wok and heat to boiling, stirring constantly, until sauce clears and thickens, about 1 minute. Stir in beef and pepper. Reduce heat to low and simmer 1 minute longer.

260   STIR-FRIED BEEF AND BLUE CHEESE SALAD

Prep: 10 minutes   Cook: 4 to 6 minutes   Serves: 3

When your dinner menus become jaded and you want something unique and easy, opt for this delicious stir-fry salad. It's designed for blue cheese lovers.

½ pound boneless top sirloin steak
2 tablespoons vegetable oil
½ pound fresh mushrooms, sliced
¼ cup chopped red onion
2 tablespoons red wine vinegar
1 tablespoon Dijon mustard

¼ teaspoon garlic salt
¼ teaspoon pepper
1 medium tomato, chopped (½ cup)
¼ cup crumbled blue cheese
½ head red leaf or romaine lettuce, separated into leaves

1. Cut beef across grain into thin strips. In a wok or large skillet, heat 1 tablespoon oil until very hot. Add beef and stir-fry over high heat for 2 to 3 minutes, until beef is browned outside but still pink inside. Remove to a plate.

2. Add remaining 1 tablespoon oil to wok and heat until hot. Add mushrooms and red onion and stir-fry 2 to 3 minutes, or until onion is tender. Add vinegar, mustard, garlic salt, pepper, and tomato and toss to blend well.

3. Return sautéed beef to wok and add blue cheese. Toss to mix. Serve immediately on individual lettuce-lined plates.

261   SWEET-AND-SOUR CHICKEN WITH PINEAPPLE

Prep: 15 minutes   Cook: 10 to 14 minutes   Serves: 4 to 6

An old-time favorite, this dish is a classy enough offering for company. It's a cinch to prepare, too. Serve with hot cooked rice.

1½ pounds skinless, boneless chicken breast halves
3 tablespoons vegetable oil
1 large onion, cut into thin wedges
1 large green bell pepper, cut into ¾-inch squares
2 tablespoons red wine vinegar

1 tablespoon cornstarch
1 (20-ounce) can unsweetened pineapple chunks, juice reserved
2 tablespoons brown sugar
2 tablespoons ketchup
1 large tomato, cut into eighths
Salt

1. Using a sharp knife, cut chicken into strips or 1-inch squares. In a wok, heat 1 tablespoon cooking oil until very hot. Add onion and green pepper and stir-fry over high heat until vegetables are crisp-tender, 2 to 3 minutes. Remove to a dish and set aside.

2. Heat remaining 2 tablespoons oil until very hot. Add chicken pieces and stir-fry over high heat until chicken is white throughout, 5 to 7 minutes.

3. Mix vinegar and cornstarch; combine with juice drained from pineapple, brown sugar, and ketchup. Add to wok. Cook, stirring constantly, until sauce clears, boils, and thickens, 1 to 2 minutes. Return onions and green pepper to skillet. Stir in pineapple chunks. Cover and cook 2 minutes longer, until heated through. Stir in tomato. Season to taste with salt.

---

262 CASHEW CHICKEN
Prep: 15 minutes   Cook: 8 to 10 minutes   Serves: 4

If you like chicken and cashews, this is a dish you won't want to miss.

6 skinless, boneless chicken breast halves, partially frozen
¼ teaspoon salt
1 large garlic clove, crushed through a press
1 egg white
2 tablespoons cornstarch
3½ tablespoons peanut or corn oil
1 red bell pepper, cut into ½-inch squares
1 green bell pepper, cut into ½-inch squares
1 bunch scallions, sliced (about 1 cup)
1 (8-ounce) can sliced water chestnuts, drained
2 tablespoons hoisin sauce
2 tablespoons dry sherry
½ cup chicken broth
1 or 2 teaspoons chili paste with garlic
¾ cup roasted cashew nuts

1. Cut partially frozen chicken into ½-inch dice. In a medium bowl, combine chicken with salt, garlic, egg white, and cornstarch. Toss to coat evenly.

2. In a wok or 10-inch skillet, heat 2 tablespoons oil over high heat until very hot. Add chicken and stir-fry until chicken is white throughout, 3 to 4 minutes. Remove chicken to a plate.

3. Heat remaining 1½ tablespoons oil in wok. Add red and green peppers, scallions, and water chestnuts. Stir-fry until crisp-tender, about 2 minutes. Remove to plate with chicken.

4. Add hoisin sauce, sherry, chicken broth, and chili paste with garlic to wok. Cook over low heat, stirring, 2 minutes. Increase heat to high and return chicken and vegetables to wok. Stir-fry, 1 to 2 minutes, or until heated through. Stir in cashews.

263   STIR-FRY CHICKEN FAJITAS
Prep: 10 minutes   Marinate: 1 hour   Cook: 7 to 10 minutes
Serves: 6

This is the way to make fajitas in a jiffy. They taste terrific. Serve with warm flour tortillas, shredded cheese, sour cream, and guacamole for a dinner hit.

5 tablespoons vegetable oil
¼ cup fresh lime juice
½ teaspoon ground cumin
⅛ teaspoon cayenne
1 pound skinless, boneless chicken breasts, cut into thin strips
1 large red bell pepper, cut into thin strips

1 large yellow bell pepper, cut into thin strips
1 large green bell pepper, cut into thin strips
1 onion, thinly sliced
1 garlic clove, minced
¼ teaspoon pepper

1. In a glass dish, mix together 2 tablespoons oil, the lime juice, cumin, and cayenne. Add chicken and toss to coat completely with marinade. Marinate chicken in refrigerator 1 to 2 hours for extra flavor, if time allows.

2. In a wok, heat 1 tablespoon oil until very hot. Add chicken with marinade and stir-fry over high heat until chicken is white throughout, 3 to 5 minutes. Remove to a plate.

3. Add remaining 2 tablespoons oil to wok and heat until very hot. Add peppers, onion, and garlic; stir-fry until crisp-tender, 3 to 5 minutes. Return chicken to wok and season with pepper. Toss until heated through, about 1 minute.

STIR-FRY BEEF FAJITAS

Increase ground cumin to ¾ teaspoon and cayenne to ¼ teaspoon. Use 1 pound flank steak, cut diagonally across the grain into thin strips, instead of chicken. Proceed as recipe directs above.

STIR-FRY SHRIMP FAJITAS

Use several dashes of hot pepper sauce instead of cayenne. Use 1 pound shelled and deveined medium shrimp instead of chicken. Proceed as recipe directs above.

264   EAST-WEST PAPAYA CHICKEN
Prep: 10 minutes   Cook: 9 to 13 minutes   Serves: 4

This is so simple and simply delicious. Serve over hot cooked rice.

3   tablespoons vegetable oil
6   skinless, boneless chicken
       breast halves, cut into
       thin strips
2   celery ribs, chopped
4   scallions, chopped
1   medium red bell pepper, cut
       into thin strips

1   firm ripe papaya, peeled,
       seeded, and cut into
       1-inch strips
1   tablespoon soy sauce
    Juice of 2 limes

1. In a wok or a 10-inch skillet, heat 2 tablespoons oil over high heat until hot. Add chicken and stir-fry until golden and cooked through, 5 to 7 minutes. Remove chicken and any drippings to a dish.

2. In same wok, heat remaining 1 tablespoon oil over high heat until hot. Add celery, scallions, and red pepper and stir-fry 2 to 3 minutes, until red pepper is crisp-tender. Add papaya, soy sauce, lime juice, and chicken. Stir-fry 2 to 3 minutes longer, until hot.

265   NECTARINE CHICKEN CURRY
Prep: 15 minutes   Cook: 12 to 15 minutes   Serves: 4 to 5

The fresh nectarines of summer add refreshing appeal to this unusual dish. Pass condiments of shredded coconut, chutney, peanuts, and raisins.

1   pound skinless, boneless
       chicken breasts
2   tablespoons vegetable oil
1   onion, chopped
3   celery ribs, chopped
4   firm ripe nectarines,
       unpeeled and sliced
1   garlic clove, minced

2½ teaspoons Madras curry
       powder
½   cup chicken broth
2   tablespoons fresh lemon
       juice
1   tablespoon cornstarch
    Pinch of sugar

1. Remove any tendons from chicken and cut into bite-size pieces.

2. In a wok or large skillet, heat 1 tablespoon oil until very hot. Add chicken and cook over high heat, stirring frequently, until chicken turns white and is cooked through, 3 to 4 minutes. Remove to a plate.

3. Add remaining 1 tablespoon oil to wok and, when hot, add onion, celery, nectarines, and garlic. Stir-fry about 5 minutes, until onion is tender.

4. Add curry powder and cook 30 seconds. Combine chicken broth, lemon juice, cornstarch, and sugar; stir to blend well. Add to wok. Cook, stirring, until sauce boils and thickens, 3 to 5 minutes.

5. Return chicken to wok and cook, tossing, until heated through, 1 to 2 minutes. Serve atop hot cooked rice.

266   APRICOT-GLAZED CHICKEN AND CARROTS

Prep: 10 minutes   Cook: 10 minutes   Serves: 4 to 5

Glaze chicken, carrots, and green beans with apricot jam for this tasty creation.

3 tablespoons vegetable oil
1 pound skinless, boneless chicken (white or dark meat), cut into ¾-inch cubes or strips
½ pound frozen green beans, thawed and drained
1 (16-ounce) package frozen baby carrots, thawed and drained

½ pound fresh mushrooms, sliced
½ cup apricot jam or preserves
1 teaspoon garlic powder
2 tablespoons red or white wine vinegar
2 tablespoons dry sherry
1 tablespoon Dijon mustard
Few dashes of cayenne
Salt

1. In a wok or large skillet, heat 1 tablespoon oil until hot. Add chicken and stir-fry over high heat 3 to 5 minutes, until chicken turns white and is cooked through. Remove to a plate.

2. Add remaining 2 tablespoons oil to wok and, when hot, add green beans, carrots, and mushrooms. Stir-fry 4 to 5 minutes, until mushrooms are softened.

3. Add jam, garlic powder, vinegar, sherry, mustard, and cayenne. Cook, stirring, a few minutes, until mixture is hot and vegetables are glazed with sauce. Return chicken to wok and heat through. Season with salt. Serve over hot cooked wild and white rice.

267   CHICKEN AND VEGETABLE PESTO STIR-FRY

Prep: 10 minutes   Cook: 10 minutes   Serves: 4

This is a hurry-up dish that is really fast. Use store-bought pesto sauce, if desired. Serve over pasta, with a bowl of grated Parmesan cheese on the side.

2 tablespoons vegetable oil
1 pound skinless chicken breast tenders
½ pound fresh mushrooms, sliced
3 cups 1-inch broccoli florets
4 carrots, peeled and thinly sliced diagonally

3 tablespoons pesto sauce (store-bought or homemade)
3 tablespoons chopped fresh basil

1. In a wok, heat 1 tablespoon oil until very hot. Add chicken and stir-fry 2 to 3 minutes, or until chicken turns white throughout. Remove chicken to a dish.

2. Add remaining 1 tablespoon oil to wok and heat until hot. Add mushrooms, broccoli, and carrots. Stir-fry until vegetables are crisp-tender, about 5 minutes.

3. Return chicken to pan. Stir in pesto sauce. Heat until hot. Add fresh basil and toss.

SALMON-PESTO STIR-FRY

Use 1 to 1½ pounds salmon steaks in place of chicken. Cook salmon steaks in hot oil in wok on both sides until cooked through and tinged with a little color, 8 to 10 minutes. Remove to dish, cover with foil, and keep warm. Proceed as directed above. Stir in pesto sauce and fresh basil before returning salmon to skillet to heat through.

---

268 CHICKEN ASPARAGUS STIR-FRY
Prep: 10 minutes   Cook: 15 to 20 minutes   Serves: 4 to 5

When fresh asparagus is in season, here's a good way to bring out its wonderful flavor and texture. Serve over rice.

1 tablespoon soy sauce	1 bunch scallions, chopped
1 tablespoon dry sherry	(about 1 cup)
1 tablespoon cornstarch	1 medium red bell pepper, cut
2 teaspoons powdered	into thin 2-inch-long
chicken flavor bouillon	strips
base	1 (8-ounce) can sliced water
½ teaspoon sugar	chestnuts, drained
1½ pounds skinless, boneless	¾ cup water
chicken breast halves, cut	¼ teaspoon salt
into 1-inch cubes	¼ teaspoon pepper
5 tablespoons vegetable oil	
1½ pounds fresh asparagus,	
diagonally sliced into	
1-inch pieces	

1. In a medium bowl, mix together soy sauce, sherry, cornstarch, bouillon, and sugar. Add chicken pieces and mix well.

2. Meanwhile in a wok or 10-inch skillet, heat 3 tablespoons oil over medium-high heat until hot. Add asparagus, scallions, and red pepper and stir-fry until vegetables are crisp-tender, 5 to 7 minutes. Remove from pan and set aside.

3. In same wok, heat remaining 2 tablespoons oil over high heat until hot. Add chicken mixture. Stir-fry, scraping bottom of wok often, until chicken turns white, 6 to 8 minutes. Stir in water chestnuts, water, salt, and pepper. Continue to cook over medium-high heat, stirring, 2 to 3 minutes, until sauce boils and thickens. Return vegetables to wok and cook, stirring, 2 to 3 minutes longer, until hot.

269 STIR-FRIED CHICKEN WITH TOMATILLOS AND PAPAYA
Prep: 10 minutes   Cook: 6 to 11 minutes   Serves: 4

Fruit salsas are in vogue for serving alongside poultry, meats, and fish. Here the salsa has been incorporated right into the recipe to give extra flavor and flair. This variation is delicious and was a hit with all who tasted. Tomatillos are green tomatoes surrounded with a brown papery husk. They are often available fresh in supermarket produce sections.

1 tablespoon vegetable oil	1 tablespoon rice vinegar
1 pound skinless, boneless chicken breast halves	2 tablespoons lime juice
	¼ teaspoon garlic powder
5 tomatillos, husked, cored, and chopped, or 1 (16-ounce) can, drained and chopped	2 tablespoons chopped Anaheim (green) chilies
	½ teaspoon salt
	1 large ripe papaya, peeled, seeded, and chopped
½ red bell pepper, chopped	
3 scallions, chopped	
2 tablespoons finely chopped fresh cilantro	

1. In a wok or large skillet, heat oil until very hot. Add chicken and stir-fry 2 to 3 minutes, or until chicken turns white throughout. Remove chicken.

2. Add tomatillos, red pepper, and scallions to wok and stir-fry 3 to 5 minutes, until pepper is tender. Stir in cilantro, rice vinegar, lime juice, garlic powder, chiles, and salt.

3. Return chicken to wok and add papaya. Stir-fry 1 to 2 minutes, until heated through.

270 SWEET-AND-SOUR WALNUT CHICKEN
Prep: 20 minutes   Cook: 10 to 15 minutes   Serves: 4

5 tablespoons vegetable oil	1 (6-ounce) package frozen Chinese pea pods, thawed
½ cup walnuts	
6 skinless, boneless chicken breast halves, cut into thin strips	3 garlic cloves, minced
	½ cup ketchup
1 medium red bell pepper, cut into thin strips	1½ tablespoons soy sauce
	1 tablespoon Worcestershire sauce
1 medium green bell pepper, cut into thin strips	½ teaspoon sugar
4 carrots, peeled and cut into thin 1-inch-long strips	1½ teaspoons Asian sesame oil
	⅓ cup water
4 scallions, chopped	

1. In a wok or 10-inch skillet, heat 2 tablespoons oil over medium-high heat until hot. Add walnuts and stir-fry until they begin to color, 30 to 60 seconds. Remove with slotted spoon to a small dish. Drain off and discard oil.

2. Add 2 tablespoons oil to wok and heat until hot. Add chicken and stir-fry until chicken is white throughout, 3 to 5 minutes. Remove to a plate.

3. Add remaining 1 tablespoon oil to wok and heat until hot. Add red and green peppers, carrots, and scallions. Stir-fry until carrots are crisp-tender, 3 to 4 minutes. Add pea pods and garlic and stir-fry 1 to 2 minutes, until pea pods are crisp-tender and garlic is fragrant.

4. Stir in ketchup, soy sauce, Worcestershire sauce, sugar, sesame oil, and water. Heat to boiling, stirring, over high heat. Boil 1 minute. Stir in chicken and heat through, about 1 minute. Stir in walnuts.

271 MOO SHU CHICKEN WITH TORTILLAS
Prep: 15 minutes   Cook: 7 to 8 minutes   Serves: 2 to 3

Moo shu chicken or pork is generally served in Chinese restaurants with paper-thin Mandarin pancakes. To save time, roll the chicken mixture in warm flour tortillas spread with hoisin sauce. While this version may not be authentic, it's mighty tasty.

½ **pound skinless, boneless chicken breasts, cut into very thin strips**
3 **tablespoons soy sauce**
1 **tablespoon cornstarch**
¼ **teaspoon pepper**
2 **tablespoons vegetable oil**
2 **cups finely shredded green cabbage**
⅓ **cup chopped bean sprouts**
3 **tablespoons chopped bamboo shoots**
2 **scallions, chopped**

4 **large fresh mushrooms, sliced**
¼ **cup chopped water chestnuts**
1 **egg, beaten**
2 **tablespoons dry sherry**
½ **teaspoon sugar**
1 **teaspoon chicken bouillon granules**
½ **teaspoon Asian sesame oil**
3 **tablespoons hoisin sauce**
4 **(6½- or 7-inch) flour tortillas, warmed**

1. In a small bowl, combine chicken with 1 tablespoon soy sauce, the cornstarch, and the pepper.

2. In a wok or 10-inch skillet, heat oil over high heat until hot. Add chicken mixture and stir-fry until chicken turns white, about 3 minutes.

3. Add cabbage, bean sprouts, bamboo shoots, scallions, mushrooms, and water chestnuts to wok. Stir-fry 2 minutes. Add beaten egg and stir-fry 1 to 1½ minutes, until egg is just scrambled.

4. Add remaining 2 tablespoons soy sauce, sherry, sugar, bouillon granules, sesame oil, and 1 tablespoon hoisin sauce to wok. Stir-fry 1 minute.

5. Brush centers of heated tortillas with remaining 2 tablespoons hoisin sauce. Spoon chicken mixture down center of each. Fold in sides of tortillas. Fold bottom quarter of tortilla up over filling, then roll up to enclose. Serve immediately with additional hoisin sauce for dipping, if desired.

272   SZECHUAN SHREDDED CHICKEN
Prep: 15 minutes   Cook: 5 to 8 minutes   Serves: 4 to 5

This dish is one of my favorites. It's not difficult to prepare, but takes a little time to assemble all the ingredients. Feel free to add vegetables as desired. Serve with rice and a fruit salad.

6 skinless, boneless chicken breast halves, partially frozen	¼ cup chicken broth
	3 tablespoons vegetable oil
1½ tablespoons cornstarch	1 medium red bell pepper, cut into thin strips
1 egg white	1 medium green bell pepper, cut into thin strips
½ teaspoon salt	
2 tablespoons hoisin sauce	5 scallions, cut into ½-inch pieces
1 tablespoon soy sauce	
1 tablespoon dry sherry	½ cup coarsely chopped bean sprouts
1 to 1½ tablespoons chili paste with garlic	¼ cup finely sliced celery or bamboo shoots
2 garlic cloves, minced	
1 tablespoon white wine vinegar	¼ pound fresh mushrooms, sliced
½ teaspoon minced fresh ginger	

1. Slice partially frozen chicken into thin strips. In a small bowl, blend cornstarch with egg white and salt. Add chicken and toss until well coated; set aside.

2. In another small bowl, combine hoisin sauce, soy sauce, sherry, chili paste with garlic, garlic, vinegar, ginger, and chicken broth; set sauce aside.

3. In a wok or 10-inch skillet, heat 2 tablespoons oil over high heat until hot. Add chicken and stir-fry until meat is white throughout and tender, 3 to 4 minutes. Remove chicken to a plate.

4. In same wok, heat remaining 1 tablespoon oil over high heat until hot. Add red and green peppers, scallions, bean sprouts, celery, and mushrooms. Stir-fry 2 minutes.

5. Return chicken to wok. Add reserved sauce and cook, stirring, until sauce boils and thickens, 1 to 2 minutes. Serve immediately.

273 THREE-INGREDIENT TASTES
Prep: 20 minutes   Cook: 10 to 16 minutes   Serves: 4 to 5

Some variation of this dish is popular on menus in many Chinese restaurants. Although the ingredient list appears lengthy, the recipe doesn't take long to put together once you've assembled all of the ingredients.

2 skinless, boneless chicken breast halves, partially frozen
½ pound boneless top sirloin steak, partially frozen
¼ pound medium or large shrimp, shelled and deveined
1 egg white
1 teaspoon salt
2½ tablespoons cornstarch
2 tablespoons dry sherry
2 tablespoons dark soy sauce
½ cup chicken broth

½ teaspoon sugar
1 tablespoon cold water
5 tablespoons vegetable oil
16 broccoli flowerets (leave 3-inch stems)
1 (8-ounce) can sliced water chestnuts, drained
¼ cup bamboo shoots
1 cup diagonally sliced bok choy
½ cup sliced fresh mushrooms
3 scallions, chopped
½ teaspoon grated fresh ginger

1. Cut partially frozen chicken into very thin strips and beef into thin slices. In a medium bowl, combine chicken, beef, and shrimp. Add egg white, salt, and 1½ tablespoons cornstarch. Using a fork, toss to mix well.

2. In a small bowl, combine sherry, soy sauce, chicken broth, and sugar with remaining 1 tablespoon cornstarch dissolved in cold water. Set sauce aside.

3. In a wok or 10-inch skillet, heat 2 tablespoons oil over high heat until very hot. Add chicken, beef, and shrimp in 2 batches. Stir-fry 3 to 4 minutes, or until cooked through. Remove to a dish.

4. Heat 2 tablespoons oil in same wok over medium-high heat. Add broccoli, water chestnuts, bamboo shoots, and bok choy. Stir-fry until broccoli and bok choy are tender, 2 to 4 minutes. Remove to dish with meat.

5. Heat remaining 1 tablespoon oil in wok until hot. Add mushrooms, scallions, and ginger. Stir-fry until mushrooms begin to soften and ginger is fragrant, 1 to 2 minutes.

6. Return meat and vegetables to wok. Stir reserved sauce and add to mixture in wok. Cook, stirring constantly, over high heat, until sauce boils and thickens, 1 to 2 minutes.

274   CHICKEN WITH PINEAPPLE SALSA
Prep: 10 minutes   Cook: 10 minutes   Serves: 4 to 5

With salsas all the rage, here's a way to incorporate a pineapple version into a stir-fry dish. This has become a favorite. Serve over rice.

3 **tablespoons vegetable oil**	3 **tablespoons chopped fresh**
6 **skinless, boneless chicken**	**basil, or 1 teaspoon dried**
breast halves, cut into	1 **tablespoon chopped fresh**
thin strips	**cilantro**
⅔ **cup chopped red onions**	1 **teaspoon dried mint**
1 **red bell pepper, chopped**	2 **tablespoons white wine**
1 **green bell pepper, chopped**	**vinegar**
1 **garlic clove, crushed**	½ **teaspoon salt**
through a press	1 **tablespoon cornstarch**
1 **medium tomato, chopped**	1 **(20-ounce) can unsweetened**
1 **or 2 green Anaheim chiles,**	**pineapple chunks, juice**
finely chopped	**reserved**

1. In a wok or 10-inch skillet, heat 2 tablespoons oil over high heat until very hot. Add chicken and stir-fry until chicken turns white, 3 to 4 minutes. Remove to a plate.

2. Heat remaining 1 tablespoon oil in wok until very hot. Add red onions and peppers and stir-fry until crisp-tender, about 3 minutes.

3. Add garlic, tomato, chiles, basil, cilantro, mint, vinegar, and salt to vegetables in wok. Dissolve cornstarch in ⅓ cup reserved pineapple juice. Stir into sauce. Cut pineapple chunks in half and add to wok along with remaining juice. Heat mixture to boiling, stirring constantly, about 2 minutes. Cook, stirring, until mixture clears and thickens, 1 minute longer. Return chicken to wok and stir in to heat through.

275   SPICY CHICKEN AND SHRIMP
Prep: 15 minutes   Cook: 6 to 7 minutes   Serves: 3 to 4

This dish is a mélange of both shrimp and chicken breast pieces along with green pepper, scallions, and garlic in a hoisin sauce mixture. Be sure to serve with plenty of hot steamed rice.

¼ **pound medium shrimp,**	1 **small green bell pepper, cut**
shelled and deveined	**into ¾-inch squares**
½ **pound skinless, boneless**	¼ **cup soy sauce**
chicken breast halves, cut	2 **tablespoons hoisin sauce**
into bite-size pieces	1 **tablespoon brown sugar**
2½ **tablespoons cornstarch**	1 **garlic clove, minced**
¼ **teaspoon pepper**	1 **teaspoon grated fresh ginger**
¼ **cup peanut oil**	¼ **cup chicken broth**
2 **scallions, chopped**	1 **tablespoon cold water**

1. Mix shrimp and chicken with 1½ tablespoons cornstarch and pepper; set aside.

2. In a wok or 10-inch skillet, heat oil over high heat until hot. Add shrimp and chicken and stir-fry until shrimp is pink and loosely curled and chicken is white throughout, 2 to 3 minutes. Remove with a slotted spoon to a plate and drain.

3. Drain off and discard all but 2 tablespoons oil from wok. Add scallions and green pepper and stir-fry over high heat 1 minute. Add soy sauce, hoisin sauce, brown sugar, garlic, ginger, and broth. Stir 1 minute. Return shrimp and chicken to wok.

4. Dissolve remaining 1 tablespoon cornstarch in cold water and stir into wok. Cook over high heat, stirring, until sauce boils and thickens, about 2 minutes. Serve immediately.

---

276 STIR-FRIED TURKEY, BRUSSELS SPROUTS, AND CAULIFLOWER
Prep: 10 minutes   Cook: 15 to 20 minutes   Serves: 4 to 5

You'll be amazed at this delicious combination of ingredients. Those who don't like Brussels sprouts may even find them tolerable in this interesting dish.

3 tablespoons vegetable oil	½ red bell pepper, chopped
¾ pound turkey tenderloin, cut into thin strips	½ cup cold chicken broth
¼ teaspoon garlic powder	1 tablespoon cornstarch
¾ pound Brussels sprouts	3 tablespoons soy sauce
½ large head cauliflower, cut up into florets	2 tablespoons dry sherry
2 celery ribs, chopped	1 teaspoon finely chopped fresh ginger

1. In a wok or large skillet, heat 2 tablespoons oil over high heat until hot. Add turkey and sprinkle with garlic powder. Stir-fry until tinged golden, 4 to 6 minutes. Remove to a plate.

2. Add remaining 1 tablespoon oil to wok. Stir in Brussels sprouts, cauliflower, celery, and red pepper. Stir-fry over high heat 5 to 6 minutes. Add 3 tablespoons water, cover, and steam over medium heat about 5 minutes, or until crisp-tender.

3. Stir together broth and cornstarch. Add to wok along with soy sauce, sherry, and ginger. Heat to boiling, stirring constantly. Cook, stirring, until sauce clears and thickens. Return turkey to pan and stir in. Heat through. Serve over hot cooked rice.

277   ORANGE-RASPBERRY-SAUCED TURKEY
Prep: 10 minutes   Cook: 5 minutes   Serves: 4

For an elegant but easy entrée, try this when fresh raspberries are in season. Serve with a hot cooked wild and white rice mixture and a tossed green vegetable salad.

2 tablespoons butter or
  vegetable oil
1 pound turkey fillets, cut into
  thin strips
1 tablespoon cornstarch
¾ cup orange juice
2 tablespoons red wine
  vinegar
1 tablespoon brown sugar

1 tablespoon raspberry-
  flavored liqueur
  (Chambord) (optional)
1 (8-ounce) can mandarin
  orange segments, well
  drained
½ pint fresh raspberries,
  rinsed and drained

1. In a wok or 10-inch skillet, melt butter over high heat. Add turkey strips and stir-fry until opaque, 3 to 4 minutes. Remove to a plate; drain excess fat from wok.

2. Mix cornstarch with orange juice; add to wok along with wine vinegar and brown sugar. Heat to boiling, stirring, until sauce clears and thickens, about 2 minutes.

3. Stir in raspberry liqueur, then gently stir in oranges, raspberries, and turkey strips. Heat through quickly.

278   STIR-FRIED PORK, SPINACH, AND NAPA CABBAGE
Prep: 10 minutes   Cook: 12 to 14 minutes   Serves: 4

If you've never tried Napa (or Chinese or celery cabbage as it's often called), which is available in many supermarkets now, here's your chance. Oval-shaped and with crinkly light green leaves, Napa cabbage is more delicate than head cabbage; it has a slight celery, peppery taste. Serve over hot steamed rice or noodles.

1 pound lean boneless pork
  loin, trimmed of excess
  fat
1 tablespoon vegetable oil
1 red bell pepper, cut into thin
  strips
1 pound fresh spinach,
  cleaned and chopped

1 head Napa or regular green
  cabbage (about 1 pound),
  shredded
1 tablespoon cornstarch
3 tablespoons chili sauce
2 tablespoons rice vinegar
1 tablespoon soy sauce
¼ teaspoon garlic powder

1. Cut pork into thin strips. In a wok or large skillet, heat oil until hot. Add pork and stir-fry over high heat until browned, about 5 minutes.

2. Add red pepper, spinach, and Napa cabbage and stir-fry 6 to 7 minutes, until spinach and cabbage are cooked down.

3. Mix cornstarch with chili sauce and rice vinegar. Add to wok along with soy sauce and garlic powder. Stir-fry until sauce clears and thickens, 1 to 2 minutes.

---

279 PLUM PORK STIR-FRY
Prep: 10 minutes   Cook: 10 minutes   Serves: 4

When fresh plums are in season, try this intriguing and flavorful dish for a change of pace.

2 tablespoons vegetable oil
1 pound boneless pork loin, trimmed of excess fat and cut into thin strips
1 large onion, chopped
1 green bell pepper, cut into thin strips
3 large firm, ripe black plums, sliced

½ cup plum jam
2 tablespoons fresh lemon juice
1 tablespoon brown sugar
½ teaspoon dry mustard
½ teaspoon ground ginger
1 tablespoon cornstarch
1 tablespoon cold water

1. In a wok or large skillet, heat oil until hot. Add pork and stir-fry over high heat until cooked through, 5 to 6 minutes. Remove pork to a plate.

2. Add onion and green pepper to drippings in wok and stir-fry just until crisp-tender, about 3 minutes.

3. Stir in plums, jam, lemon juice, brown sugar, mustard, and ginger. Heat to boiling, stirring constantly.

4. Mix cornstarch and water until blended. Stir into sauce and cook, stirring, until sauce boils and thickens. Return pork to skillet and simmer 1 to 2 minutes, until heated through. Serve over hot cooked rice.

PLUM CHICKEN STIR-FRY

Substitute 1 pound boneless, skinless chicken breasts, cut into thin strips, for pork. Stir-fry until cooked through, 3 to 5 minutes. Proceed as recipe directs.

280   HAM-ZUCCHINI STIR-FRY
Prep: 15 minutes   Cook: 8 to 10 minutes   Serves: 4

When you have plenty of baked ham on hand, this recipe is worth trying.

4 tablespoons vegetable oil	1 large onion, chopped
¾ pound baked ham, sliced ¼ inch thick, then cut into thin strips	3 tablespoons water
	½ cup chicken broth
	2 tablespoons soy sauce
3 medium zucchini, cut into ¼-inch-thick slices	2 tablespoons dry sherry
	2 garlic cloves, minced
4 carrots, cut into ¼-inch-thick slices	½ teaspoon ground ginger
	1 teaspoon sugar
1 medium red bell pepper, chopped	1 tablespoon cornstarch

1. In a wok or 10-inch skillet, heat 2 tablespoons oil over medium-high heat until hot. Add ham and stir-fry until lightly browned, 1 to 2 minutes. Remove to a plate.

2. Add remaining 2 tablespoons oil to pan and, when hot, add zucchini, carrots, red pepper, and onion. Stir-fry until onion is softened, about 3 minutes. Add water, cover, and cook 2 to 3 minutes, until carrots and red pepper are crisp-tender.

3. Meanwhile in a small bowl, stir together broth, soy sauce, sherry, garlic, ginger, sugar, and cornstarch. Stir into wok along with ham. Cook over medium heat, stirring, until mixture boils and thickens, about 2 minutes.

281   STIR-FRIED PORK WITH CHINESE VEGETABLES
Prep: 5 minutes   Cook: 10 minutes   Serves: 4

A quick-fix pork dish. Vary the vegetables according to what you have on hand in your refrigerator. Serve over hot cooked rice.

1½ tablespoons vegetable oil	3 tablespoons soy sauce
¾ to 1 pound boneless pork loin, cut into thin strips	1 tablespoon Asian sesame oil
	2 tablespoons dry sherry
4 scallions, chopped	¼ to ½ teaspoon ground ginger
1 (6-ounce) package frozen Chinese pea pods, thawed and drained	1 teaspoon cornstarch mixed with 1 tablespoon cold water
½ pound fresh bean sprouts or finely shredded cabbage	Pinch of sugar
1 (8-ounce) can sliced water chestnuts, drained	

1. In a wok or large skillet, heat vegetable oil until hot. Add pork and stir-fry over high heat until pork has no trace of pink, about 5 minutes.

2. Add scallions and pea pods to skillet and stir-fry 2 minutes. Add bean sprouts and water chestnuts and stir-fry 1 to 2 minutes.

3. Reduce heat to medium-high. Stir in soy sauce, sesame oil, sherry, ginger, cornstarch mixture, and sugar. Stir-fry until sauce boils and thickens, 1 to 2 minutes.

---

282 SPICY EGGPLANT AND PORK
Prep: 10 minutes   Cook: 20 to 25 minutes   Serves: 4

This is similar to the spicy eggplant found on menus in numerous Chinese restaurants, but in this version pork has been added.

2 **medium eggplants (about 2 pounds total), or 2 pounds small, narrow Asian eggplants**	4 **scallions, chopped**
	½ **green bell pepper, cut into thin strips**
6 **tablespoons vegetable oil**	3 **tablespoons soy sauce**
1 **pound boneless pork loin, trimmed of fat and cut into fine dice**	1 **tablespoon red wine vinegar**
	¼ to ½ **teaspoon sugar**
3 **garlic cloves, minced**	2 **teaspoons chili paste with garlic**
2 **tablespoons minced fresh ginger, or 1 teaspoon ground ginger**	½ **cup chicken broth**
	¼ **cup chopped, bottled roasted red peppers**

1. Cut unpeeled eggplant into thin 2½ × ½-inch strips.

2. In a wok or large skillet, heat 2 tablespoons oil until hot. Add half the eggplant and stir-fry over medium to medium-high heat until soft, 5 to 7 minutes. Remove to a plate and set aside. Repeat with another 2 tablespoons oil and remaining eggplant.

3. Heat remaining 2 tablespoons oil in same wok or skillet until hot. Add pork, garlic, ginger, and scallions. Stir-fry until pork is cooked through, 5 to 7 minutes. Add green pepper and stir-fry 2 minutes longer.

4. Stir in soy sauce, vinegar, sugar, chili paste with garlic, and chicken broth; cook 1 minute. Return eggplant to wok along with red peppers. Stir-fry 2 minutes to reheat. Serve with hot steamed rice.

283   COCONUT SHRIMP WITH PEA PODS
Prep: 5 minutes   Cook: 6 to 8 minutes   Serves: 4

2 tablespoons vegetable oil
1 pound medium shrimp,
   shelled and deveined
3 scallions, chopped
½ pound fresh mushrooms,
   sliced
1 (6-ounce) package frozen
   pea pods, thawed and
   drained
2 garlic cloves, minced

¼ cup canned cream of
   coconut
¼ cup cold water
1 tablespoon cornstarch
3 tablespoons dry sherry
3 tablespoons lemon juice
2 tablespoons chopped fresh
   basil
¾ teaspoon mint
½ teaspoon hot chili oil

1. In a wok or large skillet, heat 1 tablespoon oil until hot. Add shrimp and stir-fry over high heat until pink and opaque throughout, about 2 minutes. Remove to a plate (drain off any excess liquid from cooking, if necessary).

2. Add remaining 1 tablespoon oil to wok. When hot, add scallions, mushrooms, pea pods, and garlic. Stir-fry until mushrooms are tender, 3 to 5 minutes.

3. Stir in cream of coconut, water mixed with cornstarch, sherry, lemon juice, basil, mint, and chili oil. Heat to boiling, stirring, and cook until sauce thickens, about 1 minute. Return shrimp to skillet and heat through. Serve with hot cooked rice.

284   SHRIMP AND BASIL STIR-FRY
Prep: 10 minutes   Cook: 7 to 8 minutes   Serves: 4 to 5

Extend shrimp with plenty of fresh and frozen vegetables and add the flavors of pesto sauce for an interesting taste combination. Serve over rice or pasta.

3 tablespoons butter or
   margarine
¾ pound medium shrimp,
   shelled and deveined
½ teaspoon garlic powder
4 scallions, chopped
1 (16-ounce) package frozen
   broccoli, cauliflower, and
   red peppers, thawed and
   drained

1 cup frozen crinkle-cut
   carrots, thawed and
   drained
¼ pound fresh mushrooms,
   sliced
⅓ cup chopped fresh basil
2 tablespoons grated
   Parmesan or Romano
   cheese
1 large tomato, chopped

1. In a wok or large skillet, melt 1 tablespoon butter over medium-high heat. Add shrimp and garlic powder and stir-fry until shrimp is pink and loosely curled, about 2 minutes. Remove shrimp to a plate.

2. Add remaining 2 tablespoons butter to wok and, when melted, add scallions, mixed vegetables, carrots, and mushrooms. Stir-fry until vegetables are crisp-tender and hot, 4 to 5 minutes.

3. Add basil, cheese, and tomatoes. Return shrimp to pan and cook, tossing, until heated through.

---

285   KUNG PAO SHRIMP
Prep: 15 minutes   Cook: 10 minutes   Serves: 3 to 4

Wonderful looking and tasting, this hot and spicy dish made in a wok combines shrimp with water chestnuts, scallions, and a lively sauce utilizing chili paste with garlic. If you're timid about eating spicy foods, go easy on the chili paste with garlic and add less than specified in the recipe.

¾ **pound medium shrimp, shelled and deveined**
2 **tablespoons cornstarch**
1 **egg white, lightly beaten**
⅓ **cup peanut or vegetable oil**
½ **cup skinless roasted peanuts**
¼ **teaspoon crushed hot red pepper flakes**
1 **(6-ounce) package frozen Chinese pea pods, thawed**
1 **(8-ounce) can sliced water chestnuts, drained**

3 **scallions, chopped**
2 **garlic cloves, minced**
1 **to 1½ teaspoons chili paste with garlic**
¼ **cup soy sauce**
3 **tablespoons dry sherry**
1 **teaspoon red wine vinegar**
2 **teaspoons sugar**
½ **cup chicken broth**
1 **tablespoon cold water**

1. In a medium bowl, combine shrimp with 1 tablespoon cornstarch and egg white. Toss to mix thoroughly.

2. In a wok or 10-inch skillet, heat oil over high heat until hot. Add shrimp, and stir-fry until pink and loosely curled, 1 to 2 minutes. With slotted spoon, remove shrimp to a bowl.

3. Add peanuts to oil in wok and fry 30 seconds. Remove and drain on paper towels.

4. Drain off and discard all but 2 tablespoons oil from wok. Add hot pepper flakes, pea pods, water chestnuts, scallions, and garlic. Stir-fry over medium-high heat 2 minutes. Return shrimp to wok and stir-fry 1 minute longer. Mix in chili paste with garlic, soy sauce, sherry, red wine vinegar, sugar, and chicken broth until well blended.

5. Dissolve remaining 1 tablespoon cornstarch in cold water and add to wok. Cook over high heat, stirring, until sauce boils and thickens, about 2 minutes. Add peanuts and mix well. Serve immediately.

286 PINEAPPLE-SHRIMP TOSS WITH CUCUMBERS
Prep: 15 minutes   Cook: 12 to 15 minutes   Serves: 6

The combination of pineapple and cucumber may sound strange, but it works well and is delicious with shrimp in this wonderful creation.

1 pound medium to large shrimp, shelled and deveined	¼ cup red wine vinegar
	2 tablespoons ketchup
	1 tablespoon soy sauce
2 tablespoons vegetable oil	1 tablespoon brown sugar
3 scallions, chopped	1½ tablespoons cornstarch
1 red bell pepper, cut into ¾-inch cubes	1 (20-ounce) can unsweetened pineapple chunks, liquid reserved
2 large cucumbers, peeled, seeded, and cut into ½-inch dice (about 3½ cups)	

1. In a wok or large skillet, stir-fry shrimp over high heat in 1 tablespoon hot oil 2 to 3 minutes, or until shrimp turn pink and are loosely curled. Remove shrimp to a plate, draining off any excess liquid.

2. Add remaining 1 tablespoon oil to wok. When hot, add scallions, red pepper, and cucumbers. Stir-fry over high heat until pepper is crisp-tender, 3 to 5 minutes.

3. Mix together vinegar, ketchup, soy sauce, brown sugar, and cornstarch until smooth; add to wok along with liquid drained from pineapple. Heat to boiling, stirring gently, about 5 minutes, until sauce thickens.

4. Stir in pineapple chunks and shrimp. Simmer 2 minutes. Serve over hot cooked rice.

287 STIR-FRIED SCALLOPS AND VEGETABLES
Prep: 5 minutes   Cook: 12 to 17 minutes   Serves: 4

Scallops are best when cooked quickly to retain their tenderness. In this colorful dish, they are combined with assorted vegetables, and bacon adds an interesting flavor note.

1 tablespoon soy sauce	1 (6-ounce) package frozen Chinese pea pods, thawed and drained
1 tablespoon cornstarch	
1 pound sea scallops, halved if very large	
4 bacon slices, chopped	2 tablespoons water
½ pound fresh mushrooms, sliced	Freshly ground black pepper
1 medium red bell pepper, cut into thin strips	

1. In a medium bowl, mix together soy sauce and cornstarch until well blended. Add scallops and toss to coat.

2. In a wok or large skillet, cook bacon over medium heat, stirring, until crisp and brown, 5 to 7 minutes. Remove bacon and set aside. Drain off and reserve all except 1 tablespoon bacon drippings from wok. Add scallops to hot bacon drippings and stir-fry until scallops are just opaque throughout, 3 to 5 minutes. Remove scallops from pan.

3. Add 1 tablespoon bacon drippings to wok. When hot, add mushrooms, red pepper, and pea pods; stir-fry 2 to 3 minutes, or until crisp-tender. Return bacon and scallops to wok. Add water and stir-fry until hot. Season with pepper. Serve over hot cooked rice.

Chapter 10

Soup Kettle

There's nothing better to warm the soul than a steaming bowl of homemade soup. And if you add enough to the pot, a hearty soup—by itself or with one of the substantial salads in the next chapter—makes a great supper in a bowl.

Not all soups require long cooking periods. In the collection here, you'll find some winning ideas that can be cooked in a hurry, some in less than half an hour.

What makes these soups so appealing is that once everything goes in the pot, you can go about other chores, until the meal is ready to put on the table. And for the most part all you need to complete the meal is an interesting hearty bread.

Pots with nonreactive linings are favored for soup making so you don't end up with an undesirable flavored end result. Use a large pot to readily accommodate the starches, proteins, and vegetables. If you don't have one already, invest in a good-quality soup kettle or stockpot. Be sure it holds at least 10 quarts.

The soup collection here runs the gamut from Creamy Zucchini-Ham Soup to Vegetable Cheese Soup to Southwestern Chicken Soup, and much more. Kids love the Chicken and Yam Soup, Chicken Alphabet Soup, and Hamburger Vegetable Soup, to name a few. If international flavor is your choice, opt for Chicken Tortilla Soup, Hearty Beef Borscht, Tuscan Spinach Bean Soup, or Hot Gazpacho with Smoked Turkey. All rate raves in my home.

288   HEARTY BEEF BORSCHT
Prep: 15 minutes   Cook: 2 hours   Serves: 8

This Old World–inspired creation has been a mainstay in my soup repertoire for years. It's a heartwarming offering that makes a wonderful mealtime centerpiece. If you like your soup thick, use the smaller amount of water; for a thinner soup, use the larger amount. Serve with dollops of sour cream and accompany with plenty of dark bread (and butter, if your waistline allows). If you have any leftovers, refrigerate them; the soup is great reheated.

1½ to 2 pounds beef chuck roast (bone-in), trimmed of all fat
7 to 8 cups water
2 beef bouillon cubes
1 teaspoon salt
2 bay leaves
1 (12-ounce) can tomato paste
1 large onion, chopped

8 carrots, peeled and sliced
1 small head green cabbage, chopped
¼ teaspoon pepper
1 (16-ounce) can julienne-cut beets, liquid reserved (see Note)
½ cup sour cream

1. Place beef in a large soup pot. Add water, bouillon cubes, salt, and bay leaves. Heat to boiling; skim off foam. Reduce heat to low, cover, and simmer 1 hour, or until beef is almost tender.

2. Remove beef with bone and bay leaves from pot. Cut meat into bite-size pieces and return to simmering stock. Discard bones and bay leaves.

3. Stir tomato paste, onion, carrots, cabbage, and pepper into stock. Heat to boiling over high heat. Reduce heat to low, cover, and simmer 30 to 40 minutes, or until carrots are tender. Stir in beets with their liquid. Serve in large soup bowls, topped with a dollop of sour cream.

NOTE: *One bunch medium-size fresh beets (about 5), peeled and cut into thin strips, can be substituted for canned beets. Add to soup along with cabbage.*

289   BEEF AND BARLEY SOUP
Prep: 10 minutes   Cook: 1½ to 1¾ hours   Serves: 4 to 5

For a good old fashioned, soul-warming soup, try this version, reminiscent for some folks of their childhood days. It couldn't be simpler.

1½ pounds beef chuck
8 cups water
2 beef or vegetable bouillon cubes
6 carrots, peeled and chopped
1 large onion, chopped

3 large celery ribs, chopped
½ cup pearl barley
1 teaspoon salt
¼ teaspoon pepper
2 cups chopped fresh spinach or Swiss chard (optional)

1. In a 5- or 6-quart soup kettle or Dutch oven, combine beef, water, and bouillon cubes. Heat to boiling; skim off foam. Reduce heat to medium-low, cover, and simmer 1 hour.

2. Remove beef and cut into bite-size pieces, discarding any bone and fat. Return beef to pot.

3. Add carrots, onion, celery, barley, salt, and pepper. Heat to boiling. Reduce heat to medium-low, cover, and simmer for 30 to 40 minutes, until barley is tender. Stir in spinach last 15 minutes of cooking time, if desired.

---

290 OLD-FASHIONED SWEET-AND-SOUR BEEF BORSCHT WITH CABBAGE

Prep: 10 minutes   Cook: 2½ hours   Serves: 6 to 8

2 tablespoons vegetable oil
2 pounds beef short ribs, trimmed of fat
2 medium onions, chopped
2 cups thinly sliced carrots
2 garlic cloves, minced
1½ quarts water
1 (28-ounce) can crushed tomatoes with added puree

1 small head green cabbage, thinly sliced
1½ teaspoons salt
¾ teaspoon pepper
1 bay leaf
¼ cup lemon juice
¼ cup packed brown sugar
1 (8-ounce) can julienne-cut beets, drained (optional)
8 gingersnaps, crushed

1. In a large soup kettle or 5-quart Dutch oven, heat oil over high heat until hot. Add beef and cook over high heat, turning, until browned on all sides, 5 to 7 minutes. Add onions and carrots and cook, stirring often, over medium heat, 3 to 5 minutes, until onions are golden brown. Stir in garlic. Add water; heat to boiling over high heat. Skim off any residue that rises to the surface of the soup.

2. Stir in tomatoes. Reduce heat to low. Cover and simmer 1 hour.

3. Add cabbage, salt, pepper, and bay leaf. Simmer 1 hour longer. Discard bay leaf.

4. Add lemon juice, brown sugar, and drained beets. Cook over low heat 15 minutes. Stir in crushed gingersnaps.

5. Remove ribs with slotted spoon. Cut meat into small pieces; discard bones. Return meat to soup. Taste and season with additional salt and pepper to taste.

291   BEEFY SWEET-AND-SAUERKRAUT SOUP

Prep: 10 minutes   Cook: 2½ hours   Serves: 8

1 (2½-pound) bone-in beef
chuck or round steak
8 cups water
2 bay leaves
1 teaspoon peppercorns
1 (29- to 32-ounce) can or jar
sauerkraut, drained
1 (28-ounce) can cut-up,
peeled tomatoes,
undrained

1 (6-ounce) can tomato paste
¼ teaspoon salt
¼ teaspoon pepper
3 tablespoons sugar
¼ cup fresh lemon juice
1 lemon, thinly sliced

1. In a large flameproof casserole or stockpot, combine beef, water, bay leaves, and peppercorns. Heat to boiling, then skim off any residue or foam that rises to the surface. Reduce heat to low, cover, and simmer 2 hours.

2. Remove meat from pot, cool slightly, and cut meat from bone. Discard bone. Return meat to pot.

3. Add drained sauerkraut, tomatoes with their liquid, tomato paste, salt, and pepper. Mix well. Heat to boiling, reduce heat, and cook, uncovered, ½ hour. Remove bay leaves. Stir in sugar and lemon juice and heat a few minutes longer. Garnish soup with lemon slices.

292   HAMBURGER VEGETABLE SOUP

Prep: 10 minutes   Cook: 35 minutes   Serves: 5 to 6

This ranked high on the most-liked favorites list with children and teenagers who tasted it. It's great reheated, if you have any leftovers.

1 pound lean ground beef
1 onion, chopped
3 celery ribs, chopped
5 carrots, peeled and sliced
1 (28-ounce) can crushed
tomatoes with added
puree
2 cups beef broth

2 cups water
6 cups chopped Swiss chard
leaves
⅓ cup long-grain white rice
1 teaspoon basil
1 teaspoon thyme
Salt and pepper

1. In a 5-quart soup kettle or Dutch oven, cook beef and onion over medium heat, stirring occasionally, until beef is browned, 5 to 7 minutes. Drain off any fat.

2. Stir in celery and carrots and cook 3 minutes.

3. Mix in crushed tomatoes, broth, water, 3 cups Swiss chard, rice, basil, and thyme. Heat to boiling. Reduce heat to medium, cover, and simmer 15 minutes.

4. Stir in remaining 3 cups Swiss chard and salt and pepper to taste. Cover and cook 5 minutes longer.

---

293 CHICKEN TORTILLA SOUP
Prep: 10 minutes   Cook: 25 minutes   Serves: 6

This wonderful tortilla soup prepared with chicken is a meal-in-a-dish. Tasters rated it raves. It reheats well if it lasts that long!

3 tablespoons vegetable oil
6 corn tortillas, cut into thin
   strips
2 medium green bell peppers,
   chopped
1 medium red bell pepper,
   chopped
4 carrots, peeled and chopped
1 medium onion, chopped
2 garlic cloves, minced
3 skinless, boneless chicken
   breast halves, cut into
   thin strips

3 large tomatoes, peeled,
   seeded, and chopped, or
   1 (14-ounce) can peeled
   tomatoes, drained and
   coarsely chopped
1½ teaspoons ground cumin
1½ cups frozen corn kernels
6 cups chicken broth
   Juice of 1 lime
1½ cups shredded Monterey
   Jack cheese (6 ounces)

1. In a 5-quart Dutch oven, heat 2 tablespoons oil over medium-high heat until hot. Add tortilla strips and cook, stirring, until strips are crisp and golden, 2 to 3 minutes. Remove with a slotted spoon and drain on paper towels.

2. Add remaining 1 tablespoon oil to pot. Add green and red peppers, carrots, onion, garlic, and chicken. Cook, stirring often, until onion is soft and chicken is cooked through, 4 to 6 minutes. Add tomatoes, reduce heat to medium, and cook, stirring occasionally, 5 minutes. Add cumin, corn, and chicken broth. Heat to boiling, reduce heat to low, and simmer, uncovered, 10 minutes. Stir in lime juice.

3. Divide tortilla strips and grated cheese among 6 soup bowls. Ladle hot soup into bowls over cheese.

294   SOUTHWESTERN CHICKEN SOUP

Prep: 15 minutes   Cook: 1¼ hours   Serves: 6

Designed for southwestern food fans, this wonderful one-dish soup is a winner. Be sure to garnish with chopped fresh cilantro and radishes.

1 pound partially frozen skinless chicken breast tenders, chopped

2 (14 ½-ounce) cans chicken broth

3 cups water

1 large onion, chopped

5 garlic cloves, mashed

1 medium red bell pepper, chopped

½ teaspoon ground cumin

½ teaspoon oregano

1 (7-ounce) can diced green chiles

2 fresh or canned jalapeño peppers, stemmed, seeded, and minced

¼ teaspoon pepper

2 (15-ounce) cans golden hominy, drained

½ cup bottled medium-hot red salsa

6 large romaine lettuce leaves, shredded

½ teaspoon salt

½ cup chopped fresh cilantro

1 small bunch radishes (5 or 6), chopped

1. In a 6-quart Dutch oven or soup pot, combine chicken, broth, water, onion, garlic, red pepper, cumin, oregano, green chiles, jalapeño peppers, and pepper. Heat to boiling over high heat. Reduce heat to low, cover, and simmer 1 hour.

2. Add hominy, salsa, lettuce, and salt. Cover and cook over low heat 5 minutes longer. Serve garnished with cilantro and radishes.

295   CHICKEN ALPHABET SOUP

Prep: 10 minutes   Cook: 30 minutes   Serves: 4

A hearty fresh-tasting chicken, vegetable, and alphabet soup that's a relatively quick and easy meal-in-one. This is a good way to get children to eat homemade soup.

1 tablespoon vegetable oil

3 skinless, boneless chicken breast halves, cut into bite-size pieces

1 medium onion, chopped

4 carrots, peeled and chopped

3 celery ribs, chopped

1 (14 ½-ounce) can chicken broth

2 cups water

½ cup alphabets (alphabet-shaped pasta)

½ teaspoon salt

⅛ teaspoon pepper

2 cups shredded red Swiss chard or romaine lettuce

2 tablespoons dry sherry (optional)

1. In a 5-quart soup kettle or saucepan, heat oil over medium heat until hot. Add chicken and cook, stirring often, until chicken turns white; remove to a plate.

2. Add onion, carrots, and celery to pot. Cook, stirring occasionally, over medium heat, until onion is soft, 3 to 5 minutes.

3. Stir in broth, water, alphabets, salt, pepper, and chard. Heat to boiling; then reduce heat to medium-low.

4. Return chicken to pot. Simmer 15 minutes, or until alphabets and carrots are tender. Stir in sherry.

296 CHICKEN DIVAN SOUP
Prep: 15 minutes   Cook: 10 to 13 minutes   Serves: 4 to 5

For a delicious quick soup on a cool day, whip up this creation in no time.

1   tablespoon vegetable oil
2   large leeks (white and tender green), washed well and chopped
2   tablespoons flour
2   (14 ½-ounce) cans chicken broth

5   cups cut-up fresh broccoli (about 1½ pounds)
1   cup heavy cream
1½ cups shredded cheddar cheese (about 6 ounces)
1½ cups cut-up cooked chicken
¼   teaspoon white pepper

1. In a large soup kettle or Dutch oven, heat oil until hot. Add leeks and cook over medium heat, stirring occasionally, until limp, 3 to 5 minutes.

2. Stir in flour and cook 1 minute. Stir in broth and heat to boiling, stirring until thickened. Add broccoli and cook 5 to 7 minutes, until tender.

3. Stir in cream and cheese. Reduce heat to medium-low and cook 1 to 2 minutes, stirring often, until cheese is melted. Add chicken and season with white pepper. Simmer 1 minute to heat through.

NOTE: *If you don't have any cooked chicken handy, you can whip some up in the pot before cooking the leeks. Simply stir-fry cut-up raw chicken (2 to 3 skinless, boneless breast halves) in a little hot oil and remove to a dish. Add to soup as directed in recipe above.*

297   CHICKEN AND YAM SOUP
Prep: 15 minutes   Cook: 30 minutes   Serves: 4 to 5

A soup with yams may surprise you, but this one is a winner. My children were so wild about it that they asked for second helpings.

1 tablespoon vegetable oil	4 cups chicken broth
3 skinless, boneless chicken breast halves, coarsely chopped	2 cups water
	2 large yams or sweet potatoes, peeled and cut into ¾-inch pieces
1 medium onion, chopped	¼ teaspoon thyme
3 medium celery ribs, chopped	1 (10-ounce) package baby lima beans
1 small red bell pepper, chopped	½ teaspoon salt
½ teaspoon minced garlic	¼ teaspoon pepper

1. In a large soup kettle or saucepan, heat oil over high heat until hot. Add chicken and cook, stirring often, over high heat, until chicken is cooked through, 4 to 5 minutes.

2. Add onion, celery, red pepper, and garlic and cook, stirring often, 2 to 3 minutes, or until limp.

3. Stir in chicken broth, water, yams, and thyme. Heat to boiling, reduce heat to medium-low, and simmer, uncovered, 15 minutes. Add lima beans and cook 5 minutes longer, or until yams are tender. Stir in salt and pepper.

298   TURKEY SOUP
Prep: 30 minutes   Cook: 2½ hours   Serves: 8

Get the most from a whole roasted turkey by using the carcass to make this turkey soup, a one-pot meal.

1 turkey carcass	2 chicken bouillon cubes
3 to 3½ quarts cold water	¾ teaspoon salt
2 bay leaves	¼ teaspoon pepper
3 fresh parsley sprigs	½ teaspoon dried dill weed
1 large onion, chopped	1 teaspoon Worcestershire sauce
4 celery ribs, chopped	
1 cup shredded carrots	1 (10-ounce) package frozen mixed vegetables
1 cup converted rice	
1 (14 ½-ounce) can cut-up, peeled tomatoes, undrained	

1. In an 8-quart stockpot or kettle, combine turkey carcass, water to cover, bay leaves, and parsley. Heat to boiling over high heat. Skim off and discard any scum that forms on top. Reduce heat to medium-low, cover, and simmer 1½ hours.

2. Remove from heat. Remove turkey carcass. When cool enough to handle, pull off meat from bones; discard bones. Strain soup into large soup pot and discard debris. Return meat to soup. (Soup can be prepared up to this point and kept refrigerated, covered, 2 days.)

3. If soup is chilled, remove any hardened fat from top. Or skim off fat if soup is still warm.

4. Add onion, celery, carrots, rice, tomatoes, bouillon cubes, salt, pepper, dill weed, and Worcestershire sauce to soup. Heat to boiling over high heat. Reduce heat to medium-low and simmer, uncovered, stirring occasionally, 25 minutes. Stir in mixed vegetables and cook over medium heat, uncovered 5 minutes longer, or until vegetables are tender.

---

299   HOT GAZPACHO WITH SMOKED TURKEY
Prep: 20 minutes   Cook: 35 minutes   Serves: 4 to 6

Serve hot or cold as a main-dish meal. Accompany with toasted pita bread and your favorite in-season fruit.

1 (14 ½-ounce) can beef broth	¼ teaspoon salt
1 (46-ounce) can vegetable juice cocktail (such as V8 juice)	¼ to ½ teaspoon cayenne
	1 pound hickory-smoked turkey, cut into ½-inch cubes
1 small cucumber, peeled, seeded, and chopped	
1 medium green bell pepper, finely chopped	2 medium tomatoes, chopped
	6 scallions, chopped
3 garlic cloves, minced	1 (6-ounce) package seasoned salad croutons
¼ cup red wine vinegar	½ cup sour cream
2 teaspoons tarragon	6 radishes, finely chopped

1. In a 4- or 5-quart soup pot, combine broth, vegetable juice, cucumber, green pepper, garlic, vinegar, tarragon, salt, and cayenne. Mix thoroughly.

2. Heat to boiling, covered, over high heat. Reduce heat to low and simmer 20 minutes.

3. Add turkey, cover, and cook over low heat 10 minutes longer. Serve in soup bowls, topped with tomatoes, scallions, croutons, sour cream, and radishes. This soup can also be served chilled.

300   IRISH PUB SOUP
Prep: 30 minutes   Cook: 1 hour   Serves: 6 to 8

Reminiscent of the style of soup you might be served in an Irish pub, this variation is easy and delicious and will warm and comfort the soul.

1 pound bacon, cut into 1-inch pieces	2 (14½-ounce) cans beef broth
2 large carrots, peeled and sliced	1½ quarts water
½ cup chopped celery tops	1 (12-ounce) bottle ale
2 large leeks (white and tender green), washed well and thinly sliced	1 teaspoon salt
	½ teaspoon grated nutmeg
	½ teaspoon pepper
	2 cups cheddar cheese, shredded (½ pound)
4 pounds russet potatoes, peeled and cut into 1-inch cubes	½ cup chopped parsley

1. In a 6-quart soup pot, brown bacon over medium heat until crisp, 10 to 15 minutes. Remove bacon with a slotted spoon and discard all fat from pan.

2. In same pan, combine carrots, celery tops, leeks, potatoes, broth, and water. Cover and heat to boiling over high heat. Reduce heat to medium, cover, and cook 35 to 40 minutes, until all vegetables are very soft.

3. Reduce heat to low, and using an electric hand mixer on medium speed, beat together all ingredients in pot until smooth, about 5 minutes. Discard any debris that collects on beaters. (Or puree vegetables in blender or food processor.)

4. Stir in ale, salt, nutmeg, and pepper. Cover and cook over low heat 5 minutes. Just before serving, stir in cheese and parsley.

301   CREAMY ZUCCHINI-HAM SOUP
Prep: 10 minutes   Cook: 1 hour   Serves: 6

A nifty trick and the easiest way to puree the zucchini mixture is by putting an electric hand beater right into the soup pot. You avoid the mess and hassle of transferring batches to the food processor or blender.

3 pounds zucchini, cut into ½-inch slices	1 (1-pound) package frozen mixed vegetables
2 (14½-ounce) cans chicken broth	¾ pound thinly sliced cooked ham, cut into thin strips
4 cups water	1 cup light cream or half-and-half
1 cup coarsely chopped celery tops	½ teaspoon salt
9 scallions, chopped	¼ teaspoon pepper
1 medium red bell pepper, finely chopped	

1. In a 6-quart soup pot, mix together zucchini, broth, water, celery tops, and scallions. Heat to boiling over high heat. Reduce heat to medium. Cover and simmer 40 minutes.

2. Reduce heat to low. Using an electric hand mixer on low speed, beat ingredients in pot until large chunks are broken up. Increase speed on mixer and beat for 3 to 5 minutes, or until soup is thick and smooth. Discard any debris that collects on beaters. (Or puree in a blender or food processor.)

3. Stir in red pepper, mixed vegetables, ham, cream, salt, and pepper. Cover and cook over medium-low heat 10 minutes, or until vegetables are hot.

---

302   SAVOY CABBAGE MEATBALL SOUP
Prep: 40 minutes   Cook: 2 hours   Serves: 8

Here the favorite flavors of stuffed cabbage are rolled into a one-pot soup. Although the ingredient list may appear long, the recipe is not difficult to prepare and the results are well worth the effort.

1½ pounds ground turkey, pork, or veal (or a combination of the 3)
3 scallions, finely chopped
1 tart green apple, peeled, cored, and finely chopped
7 garlic cloves, minced
2 teaspoons salt
1 teaspoon pepper
1 egg
½ cup seasoned bread crumbs
2 large onions, chopped
6 carrots, peeled and thinly sliced

3 celery ribs, thinly sliced
½ pound fresh mushrooms, sliced
1½ pounds small red potatoes, scrubbed and quartered
2 (28-ounce) cans cut-up, peeled tomatoes, undrained
4 (14 ½-ounce) cans chicken broth
2 cups dry white wine
2 bay leaves
1 (1-pound) head Savoy cabbage, shredded

1. In a 6-quart Dutch oven, prepare meatballs by combining ground meat, scallions, apple, 2 of the garlic cloves, 1½ teaspoons salt, ½ teaspoon pepper, egg, and bread crumbs. Mix well with your hands and form into 2 to 2½ dozen meatballs about 1½ inches in diameter. Set aside on wax paper.

2. In same pot, prepare soup. Combine remaining garlic, onions, carrots, celery, mushrooms, potatoes, tomatoes with their liquid, broth, wine, and bay leaves. Heat to boiling over high heat. Reduce heat to low.

3. Carefully place meatballs in soup mixture. Cover and simmer 1 hour and 15 minutes. Discard bay leaves.

4. Stir in cabbage and remaining ½ teaspoon each salt and pepper. Cover and simmer 15 minutes longer.

303 LENTIL SOUP WITH SAUSAGE

Prep: 5 minutes   Cook: 1 hour 10 minutes   Serves: 4 to 6

A simple main-dish soup that goes together effortlessly with the humble lentil. Contrary to popular belief, there's no need to soak the lentils.

½ pound fully cooked Polish
    kielbasa sausage,
    quartered and sliced
1 onion, chopped
4 carrots, peeled and chopped
2 celery ribs, chopped
1½ cups dried lentils, rinsed
    and any debris discarded

6 cups water
2 bay leaves
½ teaspoon salt
¼ teaspoon pepper
2 tablespoons dry white wine
    (optional)

1. In a large flameproof casserole or soup pot, combine sausage, onion, carrots, and celery. Cook over medium heat, stirring often, 5 to 10 minutes, or until sausage browns lightly.

2. Add all remaining ingredients except wine. Heat to boiling. Reduce heat to low, cover pan, and simmer 50 to 60 minutes, or until lentils are tender.

3. Stir in wine. Cook 5 minutes longer. Remove bay leaves before serving.

304 ITALIAN SAUSAGE, ORZO, AND VEGETABLE SOUP

Prep: 15 minutes   Cook: 55 minutes   Serves: 6 to 7

Orzo is rice-shaped pasta, and it's great to toss uncooked into soups, such as this Italian-flavored one.

1 pound sweet Italian
    sausage, removed from
    casings
1 medium onion, chopped
2 garlic cloves, minced
1 (28-ounce) can crushed
    tomatoes with added
    puree
6 cups water
½ cup orzo

2 individual serving-size
    packets instant beef broth
    seasoning
1 tablespoon basil
1 teaspoon fennel seeds
1 pound fresh green beans,
    trimmed and cut into
    1-inch lengths
6 carrots, peeled and chopped
2 cups chopped zucchini
¼ cup dry white wine

1. In a large soup pot or 5-quart Dutch oven, crumble sausage and cook over medium heat, stirring often, about 10 minutes, or until well browned. Drain off all fat.

2. Add onion and garlic to pot and cook, stirring often, until onion is softened, about 3 minutes.

3. Stir in tomatoes, water, orzo, and broth seasoning. Heat to boiling over high heat, stirring occasionally. Stir in basil, fennel seeds, green beans, and carrots. Bring to a boil, reduce heat to medium-low, and simmer, uncovered, 20 to 25 minutes, until beans and carrots are almost tender. Stir in zucchini and wine and cook 5 to 10 minutes longer, or until vegetables are tender.

305   SPLIT PEA SOUP WITH HAM
Prep: 10 minutes   Cook: 1¾ hours   Serves: 8

A perfect choice for a cool-weather supper. All you need for an accompaniment is thick slices of black bread spread with butter.

1 (1-pound) package dried yellow or green split peas (or use half of each)	1 teaspoon marjoram
	½ teaspoon thyme
	1½ cups chopped carrots
1 (1-pound) piece baked ham or 1 large meaty ham bone, trimmed of fat	3 celery ribs, chopped
	¼ cup minced parsley
8 cups water	½ teaspoon salt
2 medium onions, finely chopped, plus 1 onion, peeled and studded with 2 whole cloves	½ teaspoon pepper

1. In a large stockpot or soup kettle, combine dry peas, ham, and water. Heat to boiling over high heat and skim off any residue that rises to the surface.

2. Add chopped onions and whole onion studded with cloves, marjoram, and thyme. Heat to boiling over high heat. Reduce heat to low. Simmer, covered, 1 hour.

3. Add carrots, celery, parsley, salt, and pepper. Cook, covered, over medium-low heat, until peas are very tender, about 30 minutes. Remove whole onion and ham from soup. Discard onion. Cut ham into bite-size pieces; discard any bone. Return ham to pot.

306 SAUSAGE BEAN SOUP
Prep: 10 minutes   Cook: 30 minutes   Serves: 4

Sausage lends wonderful flavor to this hearty main-dish soup, ideal for a chilly night or for any evening when nothing but a bowl of soup will suffice. Since long cooking is not required, you can make and serve this the same evening.

¾ pound fully cooked Polish
   kielbasa sausage,
   chopped
1 onion, chopped
1 teaspoon minced garlic
1 (14½-ounce) can stewed
   tomatoes, undrained
1 (16-ounce) can tomato puree
1 (10-ounce) package frozen
   chopped spinach,
   partially thawed

1 (15-ounce) can cannellini
   beans (white kidney
   beans), rinsed and
   drained
2 cups water
2 tablespoons minced fresh
   dill or 1 tablespoon dried
¼ teaspoon salt
¼ teaspoon pepper
   Dash of cayenne

1. In a large flameproof casserole or stockpot, cook sausage with onion over medium to medium-low heat, stirring often, about 10 minutes, or until lightly browned. Drain off excess fat.

2. Stir in garlic, tomatoes with their liquid, tomato puree, spinach, beans, water, dill, salt, pepper, and cayenne. Heat to boiling, stirring occasionally. Reduce heat to low and simmer, uncovered, 15 minutes.

307 QUICK CLAM CHOWDER
Prep: 10 minutes   Cook: 20 minutes   Serves: 4 to 5

On a cold winter evening, this is an easy main-dish soup to whip up. Serve with plenty of bread or rolls, a vegetable relish tray, and fruit for dessert.

2 tablespoons butter or
   margarine
1 onion, chopped
2 celery ribs, chopped
3 tablespoons flour
1 cup water
2 (6½-ounce) cans minced
   clams, liquid reserved
3 carrots, peeled and
   shredded

4 medium russet potatoes,
   peeled and cut into small
   dice
3 cups light cream, half-and-
   half, or milk
   Dash of pepper
1 teaspoon Worcestershire
   sauce
½ teaspoon dried dill weed

1. In a large saucepan, melt butter over medium heat. Add onion and celery and cook, stirring often, until onion is tender but not browned.

2. Blend in flour and cook, stirring, 2 minutes. Add water gradually and stir until water comes to a boil.

3. Add liquid drained from clams along with carrots, potatoes, light cream, and pepper. Heat to boiling, reduce heat to low, cover, and simmer until potatoes are just tender, 12 to 15 minutes.

4. Stir in clams, Worcestershire sauce, and dill weed. Simmer 2 minutes.

---

308 IN-A-HURRY FISH SOUP
Prep: 10 minutes   Cook: 45 to 50 minutes   Serves: 6 to 8

This is an easy and dependable recipe.

2 tablespoons vegetable oil
1 medium onion, sliced
¼ cup chopped fresh parsley
2 garlic cloves, minced
1 (10-ounce) can whole baby
  clams
1 bay leaf
½ teaspoon thyme
1 teaspoon salt
⅛ teaspoon pepper

2 (15-ounce) cans tomato sauce
  special (with tomato bits,
  onions, celery, and green
  peppers)
1½ pounds fresh or frozen
  halibut fillets, cut into
  chunks
1 pound medium shrimp,
  shelled and deveined
6 to 8 toasted French bread
  rounds

1. In a 4- or 5-quart pot, heat oil over medium heat until hot. Add onion, parsley, and garlic. Cook 2 to 3 minutes, until onion is soft.

2. Drain and reserve clams and clam juice. Add enough water to clam juice to measure 4 cups. Add liquid to vegetables in pot. Season with bay leaf, thyme, salt, and pepper. Heat to boiling, cover, reduce heat, and simmer 30 minutes. Remove and discard bay leaf.

3. Add tomato sauce to pot and heat to boiling over high heat. Reduce heat to low. Add halibut and simmer 8 minutes. Add shrimp and reserved clams. Simmer 5 minutes, or until fish is opaque throughout and tender.

4. Lift out halibut pieces, shrimp, and clams; arrange on a serving platter. Ladle soup into 6 to 8 individual soup plates or 1 large tureen. Lay toasted bread rounds on surface of soup. Garnish both soup and platter of fish with a sprinkling of chopped fresh parsley. Serve together.

309 EASY MINESTRONE
Prep: 15 minutes   Cook: 1¼ hours   Serves: 6 to 8

An Italian favorite, this array of vegetables in seasoned beef stock is a hearty meal-in-a-pot.

1½ pounds beef chuck,
   trimmed of all fat
1 teaspoon salt
6 cups water
1 (15-ounce) can butter beans,
   drained
1 cup ½-inch pieces fresh
   green beans
3 medium carrots, peeled and
   chopped
2 large red potatoes, peeled
   and diced
2 medium tomatoes, coarsely
   chopped

1 medium onion, chopped
2 tablespoons chopped
   parsley
1½ teaspoons basil
   Freshly ground pepper
1 small head green cabbage,
   chopped
1 (10-ounce) package frozen
   peas, partially thawed
1 large zucchini, chopped
¼ cup grated Parmesan cheese

1. In a large soup pot, combine beef, salt, water, butter beans, green beans, carrots, potatoes, tomatoes, onion, parsley, basil, and pepper. Cover and heat to boiling over high heat. Reduce heat to low and add cabbage. Cover and simmer 1 hour.

2. Remove beef from soup, cut meat into small pieces, and return to soup; discard bones. Stir in peas and zucchini. Simmer over low heat 5 to 10 minutes, until zucchini is tender. Serve topped with a sprinkling of cheese.

310 VEGETABLE CHEESE SOUP
Prep: 15 minutes   Cook: 1¼ hours   Serves: 10

Filled with lots of vegetables and covered on top with lots of cheddar cheese, all you need to complete this soup meal is plenty of garlic bread.

3 tablespoons vegetable oil
1 large onion, chopped
6 carrots, peeled and chopped
2 celery ribs, chopped
3 medium potatoes, cut into
   eighths
2 teaspoons basil
1 teaspoon oregano
1 cup tomato puree
1 (2⅝-ounce) package oxtail
   soup mix

8 cups hot water or beef broth
1 teaspoon salt
½ teaspoon pepper
2 cups fresh cauliflower florets
2 cups fresh broccoli florets
1½ cups sliced fresh
   mushrooms
3 to 4 cups shredded cheddar
   cheese (¾ to 1 pound), at
   room temperature

1. In a large stockpot or soup kettle, heat oil over medium-high heat. Add onion, carrots, and celery and cook, stirring occasionally, until onion and celery are softened, about 4 minutes.

2. Add potatoes, basil, oregano, and tomato puree. Cook, stirring, 1 minute. Add dry soup mix, water, salt, and pepper. Heat to boiling over high heat. Reduce heat to low, cover, and simmer 45 minutes.

3. Add cauliflower, broccoli, and mushrooms. Cook over medium-low heat until cauliflower is tender, about 15 minutes. Ladle soup into bowls and sprinkle top generously with cheese.

311 GARDEN VEGETABLE SOUP
Prep: 10 minutes   Cook: 25 to 30 minutes   Serves: 4 to 5

A wonderfully fresh-tasting, light soup that can be made in no time. Vary the vegetables according to your refrigerator produce bin, but be sure to use leeks—they make the dish special tasting. If desired, uncooked cut-up pieces of chicken breasts can be added the last 5 to 10 minutes of cooking time.

2 tablespoons butter	4 large red potatoes, scrubbed and coarsely chopped
2 large leeks (white and tender green), washed well and chopped	2 tomatoes, chopped
6 carrots, peeled and chopped	½ cup chopped fresh basil
1 medium red bell pepper, chopped	½ teaspoon pepper
1½ teaspoons minced garlic	Optional: 3 skinless, boneless chicken breast halves, finely chopped
3 (14½-ounce) cans chicken broth	

1. In a 5-quart soup kettle or Dutch oven, melt butter over medium heat. Add leeks, carrots, red pepper, and garlic and cook, stirring often, until crisp-tender, about 10 minutes.

2. Add broth and heat to boiling. Add potatoes, reduce heat to medium, cover, and simmer about 10 minutes, until potatoes are tender.

3. Stir in tomatoes, basil, pepper, and chicken. Cook 5 to 7 minutes longer, or until chicken is cooked through.

312　FAST TORTELLINI SOUP
Prep: 15 minutes　Cook: 20 minutes　Serves: 4 to 5

This excellent soup can be made in a jiffy. It was popular with adults and children alike.

1　tablespoon vegetable oil	1　teaspoon saltless parsley
1　medium onion, chopped	seasoning blend
2　cups chopped zucchini	2　(14½-ounce) cans chicken
(1 large)	broth
2　cups chopped carrots	1　(9-ounce) package fresh
1　teaspoon minced garlic	cheese tortellini
⅓　cup chopped fresh basil, or	2　cups frozen corn kernels
1 tablespoon dried	4　to 5 tablespoons grated
2　medium tomatoes, chopped	Parmesan or Romano
¼　teaspoon pepper	cheese (optional)

1. In a 5-quart soup kettle or Dutch oven, heat oil until hot over medium heat. Add onion, zucchini, carrots, and garlic. Cook, stirring often, until onion is limp, about 5 minutes.

2. Add basil, tomatoes, pepper, parsley seasoning blend, and broth. Heat to boiling, about 10 minutes. Stir in tortellini and corn. Reduce heat to medium and simmer until tortellini are tender, 5 to 6 minutes. Serve in bowls topped with a sprinkling of cheese, if desired.

313　CORN AND WHITE BEAN CHOWDER
Prep: 10 minutes　Cook: 20 minutes　Serves: 5 to 6

The addition of a can of white kidney beans makes a wonderful main-dish chowder to serve for supper on a chilly evening, or when you're yearning for a homey main dish.

6　thick slices bacon (about	1　(15-ounce) can cannellini
5 ounces), chopped	beans (white kidney
1　onion, chopped	beans), rinsed and
1　red bell pepper, chopped	drained
3　carrots, peeled and chopped	¼　teaspoon celery seeds
2　tablespoons flour	1　tablespoon red wine vinegar
3　cups milk or light cream	¼　teaspoon salt
1　(16-ounce) package frozen	¼　teaspoon pepper
corn kernels	

1. In a large flameproof casserole or stockpot, cook bacon over medium heat until crisp, about 7 minutes. Drain off all except 1 tablespoon drippings.

2. Stir in onion, red pepper, and carrots. Cook, stirring often, until onion is limp, about 3 minutes. Stir in flour, blending thoroughly. Cook, stirring, 1 to 2 minutes. Stir in milk and heat to boiling.

3. Mix in corn, beans, celery seeds, vinegar, salt, and pepper; heat to boiling. Reduce heat to low and simmer 5 minutes.

314   TUSCAN SPINACH BEAN SOUP

Prep: 10 minutes   Cook: 25 to 30 minutes   Serves: 6

A wonderfully hearty whole-meal soup using white beans and macaroni.

1 tablespoon olive oil
1 medium onion, chopped
2 teaspoons minced garlic
2 celery ribs, chopped
3 carrots, peeled and sliced
1 (14½-ounce) can chicken broth
1 (28-ounce) can cut-up, peeled tomatoes, undrained
½ cup small elbow macaroni
2 tablespoons chopped parsley

2 teaspoons basil
1 (15-ounce) can cannellini beans (white kidney beans), rinsed and drained
12 ounces fresh spinach, stemmed and cut up (about 4 cups)
½ teaspoon salt
½ teaspoon pepper
Grated Parmesan cheese, as accompaniment

1. In a large flameproof casserole or large soup pot, heat oil over medium heat. Add onion, garlic, celery, and carrots. Cook, stirring often, until onion is softened, 5 to 6 minutes.

2. Mix in broth, tomatoes with their liquid, macaroni, parsley, basil, beans, spinach, salt, and pepper. Heat to boiling, reduce heat to low, and simmer 15 to 20 minutes, or until macaroni is tender.

3. Serve hot, sprinkled with Parmesan cheese, if desired.

Chapter 11

Salad Bowl

When lighter fare is your choice, make a stylish meal-in-a-single-dish in a salad bowl. Everyone loves bright, tantalizing salads, brimming with the freshest, high-quality produce the season has to offer. Granted, a salad bowl is not technically a pot, but we've taken the liberty to refer to it as one because it's a utensil that can be used for creating an entire meal in one dish.

The salads on the pages that follow are designed to be served as entrées. They offer attractive, nutritious, easy, and convenient ways to get meals on the table, often without any cooking at all.

The options here are sumptuous and appealing. They combine greens, herbs, spices, vegetables, fruits, meats, fish, poultry, beans, pastas, cheeses, vinegars, and oils in myriad ways for spontaneous, original, and delicious creations.

In keeping with the one-pot theme, the dressings are often prepared in the salad bowl prior to tossing in the remaining ingredients, speeding up serving as well as cleanup chores. For best results, use glass, stainless steel, or wooden salad bowls.

Be sure the greens, vegetables, and other ingredients are dry before dressing them, because moisture dilutes the dressing. Also toss greens with dressing just before serving to keep them from wilting.

Use these recipes as blueprints to compose your own salad masterpieces. Keep in mind texture as well as composition and color. For added interest, experiment with the wide array of greens now available in many markets. Besides romaine and red and green leaf lettuces, try watercress, small mustard greens, arugula, curly endive, limestone lettuce, or even that slightly bitter red Italian leaf—radicchio.

Welcome a selection of these recipe suggestions to your table not only when the weather sizzles, but anytime when you want to get dinner on the table in a jiffy and there's no time to cook.

315 CHICKEN, RED PEPPER, AND SNOW PEA SALAD

Prep: 15 minutes   Cook: 5 minutes   Serves: 4 to 5

You can whip this together in short order if you pick up already cooked chicken at the supermarket, or have cooked chicken on hand. It's colorful, delicious, and always rates raves when served.

5 tablespoons vegetable oil
½ cup pine nuts
3 garlic cloves, minced
½ pound fresh snow peas, ends trimmed
2 large red bell peppers, cut into 1-inch pieces
2 cups cut-up cooked chicken

2 tablespoons balsamic vinegar
1 tablespoon lemon juice
2 teaspoons Asian sesame oil
¼ teaspoon salt
6 to 7 cups assorted salad greens

1. In a 3-quart pot, heat 1 tablespoon vegetable oil over medium heat. Add pine nuts and 1 minced garlic clove. Cook, stirring, until golden, 2 to 3 minutes. Remove to paper towels to drain.

2. Fill same pot three quarters full with water and heat to boiling over high heat. Add snow peas and red peppers and cook 1 to 2 minutes, until crisp-tender. Drain and rinse under cold water. Drain well; return to pot.

3. Add remaining 4 tablespoons vegetable oil and 2 minced garlic cloves to pot along with chicken, balsamic vinegar, lemon juice, sesame oil, and salt. Toss until well mixed. Refrigerate at least 1 hour or overnight before serving. Serve on a bed of greens.

316 PICNIC CHICKEN VEGETABLE BOWL

Prep: 15 minutes   Cook: none   Serves: 6

An easy and simple creation to brighten any picnic or summertime outdoor menu.

1½ pounds zucchini, chopped
4 medium tomatoes, chopped
1 (16-ounce) package frozen peas, thawed and drained
1 medium green bell pepper, chopped
1 medium yellow bell pepper, chopped

2 cups diced cooked chicken or ham
¾ cup bottled or homemade Italian dressing
3 tablespoons Parmesan cheese (optional)

1. In a large bowl, combine all ingredients. Toss to mix well. Cover and refrigerate several hours.

2. Drain and serve on lettuce.

317 CURRIED CHICKEN AND CORN SALAD
Prep: 10 minutes   Cook: none   Serves: 4

This interesting salad makes a great warm-weather dinner choice—and it's so easy!

1 cup sour cream or plain yogurt	2 cups cooked corn kernels
2 tablespoons mango chutney	1 medium green bell pepper, chopped
1 tablespoon curry powder	1 cup chopped, seeded fresh tomatoes
2 tablespoons white wine vinegar	2 scallions, chopped
¼ teaspoon salt	6 cups shredded lettuce
¼ teaspoon pepper	
2 cups shredded cooked chicken breast	

1. In a large mixing bowl, combine sour cream, chutney, curry powder, vinegar, salt, and pepper. Mix well.

2. Add chicken, corn, green pepper, tomatoes, and scallions. Toss until well mixed. Refrigerate until serving time, at least 2 hours. Serve on a bed of lettuce.

318 CHICKEN AND ROASTED PEPPERS
Prep: 15 minutes   Cook: none   Serves: 3 to 4

This is one of my daughter's very favorite quick entrée choices. If you keep a jar of roasted red peppers on hand and pick up already cooked chicken breasts at the supermarket, you can make this in a jiffy. Use fresh basil for seasoning rather than dried when it is in season.

¼ cup ketchup	⅛ teaspoon pepper
5 tablespoons red wine vinegar	2 tablespoons vegetable oil
8 ounces roasted or pickled red peppers, cut into ¾-inch pieces, liquid reserved	3 cups shredded cooked chicken breast
	¼ cup pitted ripe olive pieces
	¼ cup pimiento-stuffed green olive pieces
½ teaspoon sugar	2 tablespoons drained capers
¼ teaspoon salt	5 to 6 cups shredded lettuce
3 tablespoons chopped fresh basil, or 1 teaspoon dried	

1. In a glass bowl, combine ketchup, vinegar, and 2 tablespoons liquid reserved from roasted red peppers. Mix in sugar, salt, basil, and pepper. Whisk in oil until well blended.

2. Add chicken, red peppers, olives, and capers. Toss to mix and coat with dressing. Serve immediately or marinate 1 hour or longer in refrigerator. Serve on shredded lettuce.

319   CHUNKY CHICKEN MUSTARD SALAD

Prep: 15 minutes   Cook: none   Serves: 6

This recipe, a facsimile of an idea sampled at a take-out food establishment years ago, has become a favorite main-dish offering in my warm weather repertoire. It's a wonderful idea for outdoor picnics as well, provided it is kept well chilled.

¼ cup red wine vinegar
⅓ cup whole-grain mustard
1 tablespoon Dijon mustard
1 garlic clove, minced
½ cup vegetable oil
¼ teaspoon salt
¼ teaspoon pepper
4 cups diced cooked chicken
   breast

1 European seedless
   cucumber, unpeeled and
   diced (about 2 cups)
⅓ cup chopped red onion
⅔ cup slivered French
   cornichons or dill pickles
4 celery ribs, diagonally sliced
8 cups mixed salad greens

1. In a large bowl, combine vinegar, whole-grain mustard, Dijon mustard, garlic, oil, salt, and pepper. Mix well.

2. Add chicken, cucumber, red onion, cornichons, and celery. Toss to coat with dressing. Refrigerate at least 2 hours. Serve on greens.

320   CHICKEN SALAD NIÇOISE

Prep: 20 minutes   Cook: 10 minutes   Serves: 4 to 5

This full-meal salad is reminiscent of a traditional niçoise salad. Vary the vegetables to suit your mood and what you have handy in the refrigerator.

4 or 5 red potatoes, scrubbed
   and quartered
3 carrots, peeled and thinly
   sliced
½ pound green beans, cut into
   1-inch pieces
¼ cup red wine vinegar or
   fresh lemon juice
¼ cup light olive oil
2 teaspoons Dijon mustard
1 garlic clove, minced
¼ teaspoon pepper

2 tablespoons drained capers
¼ cup chopped fresh basil, or
   1½ teaspoons dried
2 to 3 cups shredded cooked
   chicken or turkey breast
⅓ cup thin strips roasted red
   peppers
2 scallions, chopped
1 cup ripe olives
2 hard-boiled eggs, sliced, for
   garnish

1. In a large saucepan of boiling salted water, cook potatoes and carrots 5 minutes. Add green beans and cook 5 to 7 minutes longer, or until vegetables are tender. Drain well.

2. Add vinegar, oil, mustard, garlic, pepper, capers, and basil. Toss to mix well.

3. Add chicken, red peppers, scallions, and olives. Toss until well mixed. Serve on lettuce leaves, garnished with egg slices.

321 APRICOT CHICKEN AND RICE SALAD
Prep: 15 minutes   Cook: 20 to 25 minutes   Serves: 8

4½ cups water
 1 teaspoon salt
 ½ teaspoon curry powder
 1 (1½-inch) piece fresh ginger, peeled and halved
 2 cups converted rice
 ¾ cup chopped dried apricots
 ¼ cup golden raisins
 4 scallions, finely chopped
 1 medium green bell pepper, chopped
 1 medium red bell pepper, chopped

 ⅓ cup olive or vegetable oil
 2 tablespoons white wine vinegar
 2 tablespoons dry sherry
 2 teaspoons Dijon mustard
 Pinch of cayenne
 ¼ to ½ teaspoon pepper
 2 cups diced cooked chicken breast, preferably grilled
 ⅓ cup grilled chopped toasted almonds
 Red lettuce leaves

1. In a large pot, bring water to a boil over high heat with ½ teaspoon salt, curry powder, and ginger. Stir in rice, cover tightly, and cook over low heat 20 to 25 minutes, or until water is absorbed. Discard ginger.

2. Remove rice from heat. Stir in apricots, raisins, scallions, peppers, oil, vinegar, sherry, mustard, cayenne, remaining ½ teaspoon salt, and pepper until combined. Stir in chicken and almonds. Serve immediately on red lettuce, or refrigerate and serve chilled.

322 PEA POD-PECAN CHICKEN SALAD
Prep: 10 minutes   Cook: none   Serves: 4

This wonderful salad combines chicken with pea pods, toasted pecans, and a dressing with Oriental overtones. It's great served immediately after preparation or chilled.

 3 tablespoons vegetable oil
 1 tablespoon Asian sesame oil
 2 tablespoons rice vinegar
1½ tablespoons soy sauce
 ⅛ teaspoon cayenne
 Pinch of allspice
 3 cups shredded cooked chicken breast

 4 scallions, chopped
 ½ pound frozen Chinese pea pods, thawed and drained, or ¾ pound fresh (see Note)
 ¾ cup toasted pecan halves

1. In a large bowl, combine vegetable oil, sesame oil, vinegar, soy sauce, cayenne, and allspice. Mix to blend well.

2. Add chicken, scallions, pea pods, and pecans. Toss to coat well.

NOTE: *If using fresh pea pods, trim and remove strings. Blanch in a pot of boiling water for 30 seconds.*

323   PINEAPPLE-CAULIFLOWER SALAD WITH CHICKEN AND HAM

Prep: 20 minutes   Cook: none   Serves: 6

This salad was inspired by a creation sampled at a pineapple cooking contest many years ago. Without the meat, the salad's a great accompaniment on a brunch or barbecue menu.

1 head cauliflower (about 2 pounds), cut into thin pieces (4 to 5 cups)
1 red bell pepper, chopped
1 green bell pepper, chopped
4 scallions, chopped
1 (6- or 7-ounce) can pitted ripe olives, coarsely chopped
1 (20-ounce) can unsweetened pineapple chunks, undrained

2 tablespoons red wine vinegar
¼ cup vegetable oil
¾ teaspoon salt
¼ teaspoon pepper
¾ cup chopped cooked chicken breast
¼ pound thinly sliced cooked ham, chopped (¾ cup)
5 cups mixed salad greens

1. In a large bowl, combine cauliflower, red and green peppers, scallions, and olives.

2. Drain pineapple well, reserving 2 tablespoons juice. Cut pineapple chunks in half. Add to cauliflower mixture along with reserved juice, vinegar, oil, salt, and pepper. Mix well.

3. Stir in chicken and ham. Cover and refrigerate 3 to 4 hours to blend flavors. Serve on greens.

324   SMOKED CHICKEN, WALNUT, AND GORGONZOLA SALAD

Prep: 20 minutes   Cook: none   Serves: 3 to 4

This upscale salad, similar to ones served at many restaurants nowadays, is a winner. This main-dish version contains smoked chicken or turkey, which can be purchased already cooked at many supermarkets, either in the meat or deli section. Regular cooked chicken or turkey is an acceptable substitute.

1 head romaine lettuce, washed and drained
½ head red leaf lettuce, washed and drained
¼ cup chopped fresh basil
1 cup watercress leaves
2 cups chopped cooked smoked chicken or turkey

3 tablespoons balsamic vinegar
¼ cup vegetable oil
1 cup crumbled Gorgonzola cheese
⅓ cup coarsely chopped walnuts or pecans
Freshly ground pepper

1. Tear romaine and red lettuce into bite-size pieces and place in a large salad bowl. Add basil and watercress; toss well. Keep chilled until serving time.

2. Just before serving, mix in chicken. Add vinegar and oil. Toss to coat greens well.

3. Place salad on individual serving plates. Sprinkle tops of salads with cheese and walnuts. Add a few twists of freshly ground black pepper.

325 CHICKEN-STUFFED LETTUCE
Prep: 15 minutes   Cook: none   Serves: 4 to 5

This novel main-dish salad—a hollowed-out head of iceberg lettuce filled with a chicken and cream cheese mixture—is great for a picnic or a weekend lunch. For all its good looks, it's really simple to prepare. Make it in advance and refrigerate until serving time. Serve, cut into wedges, with assorted fresh fruits and muffins.

1 head iceberg lettuce
4 ounces cream cheese, softened
⅓ cup sour cream
2 scallions, chopped
1 (4-ounce) jar pimiento pieces, drained and chopped
½ cup chopped pimiento-stuffed green olives
2 cups diced cooked chicken or turkey ham
⅓ cup chopped walnuts

1. Core lettuce, then rinse with water and drain well on paper towels. Hollow out center of lettuce (save center lettuce for use another time), making a large hole to stuff, but being sure to leave a 1- to 1½-inch lettuce shell. Refrigerate lettuce in plastic bag to crisp while making filling.

2. In a medium bowl, mix together cream cheese and sour cream until smooth. Stir in scallions, pimientos, green olives, chicken, and walnuts until well mixed.

3. Stuff mixture into center of lettuce shell, smoothing top. Wrap in plastic wrap. Chill at least 2 hours prior to serving. Cut into wedges at serving time.

326   CHINESE CHICKEN DINNER SALAD

Prep: 20 minutes   Cook: none   Serves: 6 to 8

This wonderfully attractive and simple version of the ever-popular Chinese chicken salad makes a complete main dish all by itself. Simply add rolls and fruit for dessert.

2 tablespoons Asian sesame oil
2 tablespoons soy sauce
¼ cup rice vinegar
3 tablespoons vegetable oil
1 teaspoon dry mustard
Pinch of sugar
½ small to medium head red cabbage, washed and shredded (about 4 cups)
1 head iceberg lettuce, washed and shredded (about 8 cups)

1 (6-ounce) package frozen Chinese pea pods, thawed and drained
1 (8-ounce) can sliced water chestnuts, drained
4 scallions, chopped
5 carrots, peeled and shredded (2 cups)
2 cups shredded cooked chicken (breast preferred)
Seasoned salt and pepper to taste

1. In a large salad bowl, whisk together sesame oil, soy sauce, rice vinegar, oil, dry mustard, and sugar.

2. Add cabbage, lettuce, pea pods, water chestnuts, scallions, carrots, and chicken. Toss well so salad is coated evenly with dressing. Serve immediately or refrigerate for up to 1 hour.

327   CHICKEN-PAPAYA SALSA SALAD

Prep: 15 minutes   Cook: none   Serves: 3

This salad is a winner—fabulous tasting and looking. It rates raves with all who taste. Serve on shredded red lettuce for a festive luncheon or supper offering. Accompany with warm cheese quesadilla wedges or herb-baked pita bread pieces.

1 papaya, peeled, seeded, and cut into ¾-inch cubes
½ red bell pepper, chopped
½ green bell pepper, chopped
¼ cup chopped red onion
2 tablespoons chopped fresh mint
2 tablespoons chopped fresh basil

2 tablespoons rice or white wine vinegar
1 tablespoon vegetable oil
2 tablespoons fresh lemon or lime juice
Dash of cayenne
1½ cups diced cooked chicken or turkey
5 cups mixed lettuce

In a medium bowl, combine all ingredients except salad greens. Toss to mix well. Cover and refrigerate about 2 hours to blend flavors. Serve on salad greens.

328 CASHEW, HAM, AND PEA SALAD
Prep: 10 minutes   Cook: none   Serves: 4

This take-off on an old favorite uses ham, and is great to whip up when you have more leftover ham than you know what to do with. Complete the meal with garlic bread and fresh fruit.

⅓ cup reduced-calorie mayonnaise
⅓ cup light sour cream
Juice of 1 lemon
Few drops of hot pepper sauce
1 (16-ounce) package frozen peas, thawed
1 to 1½ cups diced cooked ham

4 scallions, chopped
1 (8-ounce) can sliced water chestnuts, drained and chopped
⅔ cup roasted unsalted or salted cashews
6 cups shredded lettuce
4 to 8 large lettuce leaves

1. In a medium bowl, combine mayonnaise, sour cream, lemon juice, and hot sauce. Mix to blend well.

2. Stir in all remaining ingredients except ⅓ cup cashews and lettuce. Serve salad on a bed of shredded lettuce atop lettuce leaves. Sprinkle each salad with some of remaining cashews.

329 TABBOULEH HAM SALAD
Prep: 30 minutes   Cook: none   Serves: 4 to 6

Here's an interesting and delicious way to use leftover cooked ham in a main-dish salad. The mixture would also be good served in pita bread, sandwich style.

1 (5.25-ounce) package tabbouleh wheat salad mix
1 cup cold water
¼ cup olive oil
1 medium zucchini, chopped
1 medium tomato, chopped
3 scallions, finely chopped

1 apple, chopped
1 cucumber, peeled and chopped
½ pound leftover cooked ham, chopped
Juice of 1 lemon
6 to 8 cups shredded salad greens

1. Mix bulgur wheat and spice packet from salad mix in a large bowl. Stir in cold water and olive oil; let stand 30 minutes.

2. Add zucchini, tomato, scallions, apple, cucumber, and ham and toss with tabbouleh mixture.

3. Squeeze lemon juice over all and stir. Serve on plates lined with greens. Or serve salad in pita breads, topped with a little shredded lettuce.

330   SAVORY TURKEY SALAD ORIENTAL
Prep: 15 minutes   Cook: none   Serves: 4 to 5

This is a tasty lunch or supper offering when you prefer to dine light. Accompany with a colorful skewer of fresh seasonal fruits.

7 to 8 cups bite-size pieces of lettuce
2 cups fresh bean sprouts, or 1 (16-ounce) can bean sprouts, rinsed and well drained
1½ cups sliced fresh mushrooms
1 cup thin strips Monterey Jack cheese
1½ cups diced, cooked, hickory-smoked turkey breast
1 (8-ounce) can sliced water chestnuts, drained
4 scallions, chopped
2 tablespoons toasted sesame seeds
¼ cup vegetable oil
¼ cup rice vinegar
½ teaspoon salt
¼ teaspoon pepper
2 teaspoons soy sauce
¼ teaspoon garlic powder

1. In a large salad bowl, toss together lettuce, bean sprouts, mushrooms, cheese, turkey, water chestnuts, scallions, and sesame seeds.

2. Add oil, vinegar, salt, pepper, soy sauce, and garlic powder. Toss with lettuce mixture until well mixed. Serve immediately, or refrigerate 1 hour and serve chilled.

331   TURKEY AND BLACK BEAN SALAD
Prep: 15 minutes   Cook: 1¼ hours   Serves: 6

This salad would be a good base for a tostada salad. It would also be a good appetizer served with pita bread. Without the turkey or chicken, it makes a great accompaniment for grilled meats or fish. Serve on lettuce leaves, surrounded with chopped tomatoes and corn chips, if desired. If you cannot find red or yellow peppers, use all green.

1 cup dried black beans (8 ounces)
6 cups water
¼ cup vegetable oil
¼ cup red wine vinegar
¾ teaspoon salt
1 garlic clove, minced
Dash of crushed hot pepper flakes
¾ cup finely diced green bell pepper
¾ cup finely diced red bell pepper
¾ cup finely diced yellow bell pepper
⅓ cup finely chopped red onion
¼ cup finely chopped fresh cilantro or parsley
2 cups diced cooked smoked turkey or chicken

1. Sort through beans and discard any debris. Rinse and drain beans. In a large saucepan, combine beans and water. Heat to boiling, reduce heat to low, cover pan, and simmer 1 hour, or until beans are tender but not mushy. Drain beans and rinse with cold water. Set aside to cool.

2. When beans are cool, add all remaining ingredients. Mix well and refrigerate for 2 to 3 hours.

---

332 ARTICHOKE, HEARTS OF PALM, TURKEY, AND MUSHROOM SALAD
Prep: 15 minutes   Cook: none   Serves: 4

This is one of my salad favorites. I serve it both with and without meat for an entrée. If serving without meat, accompany with cottage cheese, a cup of soup, or a cheese-topped slice of toast.

1 (8½-ounce) can quartered artichoke hearts, rinsed and drained
1 (7½-ounce) can hearts of palm, drained and cut into ½-inch slices
2 (4½-ounce) jars sliced mushrooms, drained (see Note)
1 medium green bell pepper, cut into chunks
1 medium red bell pepper, cut into chunks

2 scallions, finely chopped
2 tablespoons drained capers
3 tablespoons red wine vinegar
3 tablespoons vegetable oil
¾ teaspoon Italian herb blend seasoning
¼ teaspoon salt
¼ teaspoon pepper
2 cups cut-up cooked smoked turkey
6 cups shredded salad greens

In a large bowl, combine artichokes, hearts of palm, mushrooms, green and red peppers, scallions, capers, vinegar, oil, Italian seasoning, salt, pepper, and turkey. Toss to mix well. Serve immediately on greens, or marinate in refrigerator several hours or overnight to blend flavors.

NOTE: *Do not use fresh mushrooms in this recipe as they will discolor the dressing and become dark if allowed to marinate for any length of time.*

---

333 ONE-BOWL TURKEY COBB SALAD
Prep: 15 minutes   Cook: none   Serves: 4

Prepare a yogurt-honey-dill dressing in the bottom of the salad bowl first, then arrange traditional cobb salad ingredients on top. Present the attractive salad untossed, then simply toss just before serving in front of diners.

1 (8-ounce) container plain yogurt	4 hard-boiled eggs, chopped
2 teaspoons honey	1½ cups fresh mushroom slices
1 teaspoon grated onion	1½ cups chopped tomatoes
½ teaspoon dried dill weed	1½ cups thin strips cooked turkey breast
⅛ teaspoon dry mustard	1 cup crisp-cooked crumbled bacon
½ teaspoon salt	
¼ teaspoon pepper	¾ cup crumbled blue or Roquefort cheese
6 cups chopped romaine or iceberg lettuce	

1. In a large salad bowl, combine yogurt, honey, onion, dill weed, mustard, salt, and pepper. Mix well.

2. Place chopped lettuce on top of dressing. Then arrange separate pie-shaped sections of eggs, mushrooms, tomatoes, turkey, bacon, and cheese on top of lettuce. Refrigerate, covered, 1 to 2 hours before serving.

3. Just before serving, toss salad, being sure to lift up and mix in dressing from bottom of bowl.

---

334 CURRIED SHRIMP SALAD
Prep: 15 minutes   Cook: none   Serves: 2 as a main dish

For an interesting main-dish salad with shrimp and cabbage, try this novel combination. A curry dressing enlivens the vegetable and shrimp mixture. Sprinkle with lightly toasted peanuts before serving.

¼ cup fresh lemon juice	2 cups shredded red cabbage
½ cup heavy cream	1 cup frozen corn kernels, cooked, drained, and cooled
4 teaspoons Dijon mustard	
3 tablespoons curry powder	
3 tablespoons sugar Generous dash of cayenne	1 cup frozen peas, cooked, drained, and cooled
5 tablespoons vegetable oil	20 cooked medium shrimp, shelled and deveined
2 cups shredded green cabbage	½ cup unsalted peanuts

1. In a large bowl, whisk together lemon juice, cream, mustard, curry powder, sugar, cayenne, and oil until well blended.

2. Add remaining ingredients except peanuts, tossing well. Serve salad, sprinkled with peanuts.

335   DILLED POTATO SALAD WITH SHRIMP
Prep: 10 minutes   Cook: 8 to 10 minutes   Serves: 4

Fresh dill in combination with bay shrimp make this refreshing salad a summer dinner favorite.

6 medium red potatoes, scrubbed and cut into 1-inch cubes	½ teaspoon salt
	¼ teaspoon pepper
1¼ cups sour cream	½ pound cooked, shelled, and deveined bay (tiny) shrimp, thawed if frozen
¼ cup red wine vinegar	
4 scallions, chopped	1 tomato, chopped (optional)
⅓ cup chopped fresh dill	

1. In a large saucepan, cook potatoes in boiling salted water until tender, 8 to 10 minutes; drain well. Transfer potatoes to a large bowl and let stand until cool.

2. Add sour cream, vinegar, scallions, dill, salt, and pepper. Stir to mix well. Stir in shrimp and tomato. Serve immediately on lettuce leaves, or refrigerate until serving time.

336   SHRIMP AND SPINACH PASTA SALAD WITH FETA CHEESE AND TOMATOES
Prep: 15 minutes   Cook: 8 to 10 minutes   Serves: 4

This appealing combination features shrimp, spinach, cucumbers, tomatoes, and feta cheese. Serve at room temperature immediately after preparing or refrigerate until chilled. Besides a light supper offering, it would be an appropriate company luncheon dish as well.

½ pound small pasta shells	2 large tomatoes, chopped
2 tablespoons balsamic vinegar	4 scallions, chopped
	1 cucumber, peeled, seeded, and chopped
3 tablespoons extra-virgin olive oil	½ pound cooked medium shrimp, shelled and deveined
1 garlic clove, minced	
1½ tablespoons Dijon mustard	½ cup crumbled feta cheese (about 4 ounces)
10 to 12 ounces fresh spinach, cleaned and stemmed, leaves shredded (5 to 6 cups)	⅓ cup toasted pine nuts

1. In a large pot of boiling salted water, cook shells until just tender, 8 to 10 minutes. Drain, then rinse with cold water and drain again. Let cool 5 minutes. Transfer to a serving bowl.

2. Add vinegar, oil, garlic, and mustard to shells. Toss well to mix.

3. Add spinach, tomatoes, scallions, cucumber, shrimp, and feta cheese. Mix thoroughly. Sprinkle toasted pine nuts over top of salad.

337   TUSCAN TUNA AND WHITE BEAN SALAD
Prep: 15 minutes   Cook: none   Serves: 2 to 3

When you need to get dinner on the table pronto, this cold dish should suffice, especially for tuna fans. My teenage daughter found this easy offering a winner.

2 large tomatoes, chopped
1 (6½- or 7-ounce) can solid white water-packed tuna, drained
3 tablespoons chopped red onion or scallions
¼ cup chopped fresh basil or parsley
2 tablespoons rinsed and drained capers
3 tablespoons red wine vinegar

1 tablespoon olive oil
¼ teaspoon garlic powder
¼ teaspoon salt
¼ teaspoon pepper
1 (15-ounce) can cannellini beans (white kidney beans), rinsed and well-drained
10 to 12 ounces fresh spinach, cleaned, dried, and torn into pieces

1. In a medium bowl, combine tomatoes, tuna, red onion, basil, capers, vinegar, olive oil, garlic powder, salt, and pepper. Mix until well blended.

2. Gently fold in beans. Serve immediately on spinach leaves, or refrigerate 1 to 2 hours before serving.

338   PINEAPPLE SEAFOOD SALAD
Prep: 15 minutes   Cook: none   Serves: 4 to 6

This unusual salad makes wonderful summertime eating. For a special presentation, serve it in hollowed-out fresh pineapple boats. You can use the cut-up fresh pineapple, if desired, but be sure to drain it well before adding to the salad mixture.

½ cup sour cream
¾ to 1 teaspoon curry powder
3 tablespoons chutney
1 tablespoon lemon juice
3 scallions, chopped
1 red bell pepper, chopped
2 celery ribs, chopped
1 (8-ounce) can sliced water chestnuts, drained
¼ cup golden seedless raisins

1 (20-ounce) can unsweetened pineapple chunks, well drained
½ pound cooked shrimp, shelled and deveined
½ pound frozen snow crab or imitation crab, thawed, rinsed, and well drained
Shredded lettuce and lettuce leaves
⅓ cup roasted cashews

1. In a medium bowl, combine sour cream, curry powder, chutney, and lemon juice. Mix to blend well.

2. Fold in all remaining ingredients except lettuce and cashews. Refrigerate at least 1 hour before serving.

3. Serve on a bed of shredded lettuce piled on lettuce leaves. Sprinkle with cashews.

---

339 ANTIPASTO SUPPER SALAD
Prep: 15 minutes   Cook: none   Serves: 6 to 8

This salad is loaded with lots of salami, cheese, garbanzo beans, tomatoes, green pepper, scallions, and sun-dried tomatoes packed in oil. It makes an ideal lunch or dinner offering when served on a bed of shredded fresh spinach or lettuce.

½ cup bottled Italian salad
    dressing
1 teaspoon Dijon mustard
3 tablespoons chopped fresh
    basil
¾ pound sliced Genoa or other
    hard salami, cut into thin
    strips
½ pound provolone cheese,
    cut into ½-inch cubes
1 (15-ounce) can garbanzo
    beans (chick-peas),
    drained

3 medium tomatoes, seeded
    and chopped
4 to 6 sun-dried tomatoes
    packed in oil, cut up
1 medium green bell pepper,
    cut into thin strips
1 bunch scallions, thinly
    sliced
½ cup ripe olive pieces
8 to 10 cups shredded fresh
    spinach

1. In a large bowl, mix together Italian dressing, mustard, and basil.

2. Add salami, cheese, beans, fresh and sun-dried tomatoes, green pepper, scallions, and olives. Toss to mix well. Refrigerate several hours to allow flavors to blend. Toss again before serving. Serve on a bed of spinach.

340 ITALIAN TWO-BEAN ENTREE SALAD
Prep: 15 minutes   Cook: none   Serves: 4

This is a great no-cook meal-in-a-dish, handy when you're in a hurry. Serve on a bed of shredded assorted greens and accompany with Italian-style bread, such as focaccia.

3 tablespoons red wine vinegar
1 tablespoon balsamic vinegar
2 tablespoons olive oil
2 garlic cloves, crushed through a press
¼ cup chopped fresh basil, or 1½ teaspoons dried
½ teaspoon salt
¼ teaspoon pepper
1 (15-ounce) can cannellini beans (white kidney beans), rinsed and drained

1 (15½-ounce) can garbanzo beans (chick-peas), rinsed and drained
1 (8½-ounce) can quartered artichoke hearts, drained
6 scallions, chopped
1 red bell pepper, chopped
1 large tomato, seeded and chopped
3 ounces thinly sliced salami, cut into thin strips
4 cups mixed salad greens

1. In a medium bowl, whisk together red wine vinegar, balsamic vinegar, olive oil, garlic, basil, salt, and pepper.

2. Gently mix in beans, artichoke hearts, scallions, red pepper, tomato, and salami. Serve immediately on a bed of mixed greens, or refrigerate until serving time.

341 BROWN RICE AND VEGETABLES
Prep: 10 minutes   Cook: 45 minutes   Serves: 4

This is a good choice for a meatless main-dish meal. Serve warm over chopped fresh spinach leaves. It's also delicious chilled.

1 cup brown rice, rinsed and drained
¼ cup olive oil
1½ cups water
2 cups frozen corn kernels
1 cup chopped carrots
½ cup frozen green peas
½ cup chopped green bell pepper

½ cup chopped red bell pepper
3 scallions, finely chopped
⅓ cup dry roasted peanuts
⅓ cup red wine vinegar
½ teaspoon garlic salt
¼ teaspoon pepper
6 cups chopped fresh spinach (about 12 ounces)

1. In a large saucepan, cook brown rice in 1 tablespoon oil over medium heat, stirring occasionally, 5 minutes. Stir in water and heat to boiling. Cover and reduce heat to low. Simmer 30 to 35 minutes, or until rice is almost tender.

2. Stir in corn, carrots, peas, and green and red peppers. Cover and cook over low heat 10 to 12 minutes, until peas and corn are cooked.

3. Stir in scallions, peanuts, vinegar, garlic salt, pepper, and remaining 3 tablespoons oil. Toss well. Serve immediately on spinach leaves.

---

342 RAVIOLI SALAD
Prep: 15 minutes   Cook: 15 minutes   Serves: 4

This novel salad uses cooked cheese ravioli. Fresh basil, if available, lends wonderful fresh flavor.

1 **(15-ounce) package frozen cheese ravioli, separated into pieces**	½ **teaspoon Dijon mustard**
2 **medium tomatoes, chopped**	¾ **teaspoon Italian seasoning**
2 **small zucchini, shredded**	½ **teaspoon minced garlic**
3 **tablespoons minced fresh basil or 1½ teaspoons dried**	¼ **teaspoon sugar**
2 **tablespoons red wine vinegar**	¼ **teaspoon salt**
	¼ **teaspoon pepper**
	¼ **cup olive oil**
	⅓ **cup grated Parmesan cheese**
	6 **cups assorted salad greens**

1. In a large pot of boiling salted water, cook ravioli until tender, about 15 minutes. Drain off water. Let cool in pan 10 minutes.

2. Add tomatoes, zucchini, basil, vinegar, mustard, Italian seasoning, garlic, sugar, salt, pepper, and olive oil. Toss gently until well mixed. Stir in cheese. Serve immediately on greens, or refrigerate 1 to 2 hours until serving.

Chapter 12

Miscellaneous Pots and Pans

This is the catch-all chapter, for all those odd pots and cooking utensils that don't fit neatly elsewhere. Here you'll find roasts and pizzas, sandwiches and tortes.

I still consider these one-pot meals, because for the most part, they all contain some type of protein, carbohydrate, and vegetable to make a complete dinner. What's even better, they'll add a little diversity and fun to mealtime.

---

343 STUFFED ROASTED CHICKEN
Prep: 10 minutes   Cook: 1½ hours   Serves: 4 to 5

This handsome and tasty stuffed roasted chicken goes together effort-lessly.

1 **(4-pound) roasting chicken**	2 **medium zucchini, shredded**
6 **scallions, chopped**	3 **cups seasoned stuffing mix**
3 **celery ribs, chopped**	**Pinch of rosemary**
⅓ **cup chopped walnuts**	⅓ **cup chicken stock**
3 **carrots, peeled and**	¼ **teaspoon garlic salt**
shredded	¼ **teaspoon pepper**

1. Preheat oven to 350°. Clean chicken, discarding giblets and neck. Rinse cavity well and remove excess fat; pat dry.

2. In a medium bowl, combine scallions, celery, walnuts, carrots, zucchini, stuffing, and rosemary. Stir in chicken stock. Toss to moisten stuffing evenly.

3. Spoon stuffing loosely into cavity and neck of chicken, pushing stuffing underneath skin near the neck. Use a metal skewer to close neck cavity; tie legs together. Wrap excess stuffing tightly in foil and set aside.

4. Season chicken with garlic salt and pepper. Place chicken, breast side up, on a rack in a foil-lined 9x13-inch baking pan. Roast 1½ hours, or until juices run clear. Place foil stuffing packet in oven during last 35 minutes of roasting time.

5. Remove stuffing from chicken and mix with stuffing in foil packet. Carve chicken and serve with stuffing.

344   CORNISH GAME HENS SUPREME
Prep: 30 minutes   Cook: 1¼ hours   Serves: 4 to 5

For easier handling by guests, remove the backbone from the hens prior to roasting on top of a vegetable-rice mixture.

4 Cornish game hens
3 tablespoons olive oil
1 carrot, peeled and chopped
1 small onion, chopped
1 (9-ounce) package brown
   and white Texmati rice
   blend with wild rice
¼ pound fresh mushrooms,
   sliced

¼ cup chopped dried apricots
¼ cup raisins
1 small green apple, cored and
   chopped
2 small zucchini, chopped
1 (14½-ounce) can chicken
   broth
½ teaspoon salt
¼ teaspoon pepper

1. Preheat oven to 350°. Rinse game hens and pat dry. Cut down both sides of backbone to remove entire backbone. Press down on breast with palm of hand to flatten each hen. Tuck wings and legs under.

2. In a large deep ovenproof baking or roasting pan (about 10x14x4 inches), heat oil over medium heat until hot. Add hens, breast side down, and cook until browned, 7 to 9 minutes. Remove hens.

3. Add carrots and onions, increase heat to high, and cook, stirring often, until onions are golden, about 3 minutes. Add rice, reduce heat to medium, and cook 2 minutes. Stir in mushrooms, apricots, raisins, apple, zucchini, broth, salt, and pepper.

4. Place hens on top of rice mixture. Cover with foil. Bake 1 hour, or until rice is tender and hens are cooked through.

345   BAKED HONEY OF A HAM
Prep: 15 minutes   Cook: 1½ to 2 hours   Serves: 10 to 12

This is an easy way to gussy up a canned ham for a holiday or anytime.

½ cup honey
¼ cup cider vinegar
¼ cup frozen orange juice
   concentrate, thawed
¼ teaspoon cinnamon
¼ teaspoon ground cloves
¼ teaspoon grated nutmeg
1 (5-pound) canned ham,
   trimmed of all gelatin and
   fat

6 medium sweet potatoes,
   yam variety, scrubbed
   well and pricked with
   tines of long fork
6 tablespoons butter
   Canned drained pineapple
   slices, maraschino
   cherries, and parsley
   sprigs, for garnish

1. Preheat oven to 325°. Combine honey, vinegar, orange juice concentrate, cinnamon, cloves, and nutmeg. Mix well.

2. Line a 10x14-inch roasting pan with a double thickness of aluminum foil.

Set rack on top of foil and place ham on rack. Pierce ham every ¾ inch with tines of a long heavy fork. Brush some of honey mixture over ham. Surround ham with sweet potatoes.

3. Bake 1½ to 2 hours, or until ham is heated through and potatoes are tender, basting ham every 15 to 20 minutes with honey mixture.

4. Let ham stand 5 to 10 minutes before carving into slices. Split open sweet potatoes and add 1 tablespoon butter to each. Serve ham slices on a platter surrounded with sweet potatoes. Garnish ham with drained pineapple slices, maraschino cherries, and parsley.

---

346 SOUTHWESTERN ROASTED TURKEY
Prep: 40 minutes   Cook: 5½ to 6½ hours   Serves: 16 to 20

When a large turkey dinner is the order of the day, try this simple version with a southwestern-inspired stuffing.

2 (12-ounce) packages seasoned stuffing mix	¾ pound fully cooked Polish kielbasa sausage, chopped
2 medium onions, chopped	
8 celery ribs, chopped	¾ cup chicken broth
1 medium red bell pepper, chopped	1 (20- to 22-pound) turkey, thawed if frozen
1 medium green bell pepper, chopped	2 to 3 tablespoons vegetable oil
1 (16-ounce) package frozen corn kernels	4 tablespoons butter, melted
1 (7-ounce) can diced green chiles	

1. In a very large bowl, combine dry stuffing, onions, celery, red and green peppers, corn, chiles, and sausage. Add broth and mix well. Stuffing will be dry, but will moisten some when baked.

2. Preheat oven to 325°. Remove giblets and neck from turkey and refrigerate for another use. Rinse turkey inside and out; pat dry. Place turkey breast side up. Stuff body and neck cavities lightly with stuffing mixture. Truss turkey. Place remaining stuffing in a large casserole dish, cover with foil, and refrigerate until baking time.

3. Rub turkey all over with oil. Place on a rack in a large roasting pan. Place in oven and roast 5½ to 6½ hours, or until done, basting with butter and pan drippings every 20 to 30 minutes. Internal thigh temperature should be 180° to 185°, and when thigh is pierced, juices should run clear. Stuffing temperature should reach at least 165°. Bake remaining casserole dish of stuffing, covered, during last hour, or until hot in center. Remove cover and continue baking another 5 to 10 minutes for drier stuffing.

4. Let turkey stand 15 to 20 minutes for easier carving. Remove stuffing from turkey and serve with turkey slices.

347 BAKED HOLIDAY FEAST
Prep: 20 minutes   Cook: 3 to 3½ hours   Serves: 10 to 12

The combination of flavors in this dish marry to make a rich, memorable meal. This is an especially good choice when time for last-minute preparations is limited. Serve with horseradish on the side.

4 pounds veal or lamb shanks
4 pounds lean meaty beef short ribs
4 pounds lean beef chuck roast or flanken, trimmed of fat and cut into large chunks
1 teaspoon salt
½ teaspoon pepper
1 teaspoon garlic powder
6 large baking potatoes, peeled

6 large sweet potatoes, peeled
6 carrots, peeled and cut into thirds
4 celery ribs, cut into 2-inch pieces
4 parsnips, peeled and cut into thirds
1 head of garlic, separated into cloves, cloves peeled
15 pitted prunes
1 cup dry white wine

1. Preheat oven to 350°. Trim meats of all fat. Place in a large roasting pan with a lid. Season with salt, pepper, and garlic powder. Cover and bake 1 hour.

2. While meat is roasting, prepare vegetables. Add potatoes, carrots, celery, and parsnips to pan. Place garlic cloves under meat and scatter prunes over top. Pour wine over all.

3. Cover and bake 2 to 2½ hours, or until meat is tender. Add additional wine or water as needed to keep mixture from drying out.

348 ROAST LEG OF LAMB WITH VEGETABLES
Prep: 10 minutes   Cook: 2 to 2¼ hours   Serves: 8

A lamb dinner is easy if you bake potatoes and vegetables in the oven alongside the meat. This is the essence of simplicity.

1 (5½-pound) whole leg of lamb
6 garlic cloves, peeled and cut in half
1 cup red pepper jelly or pimiento jam

8 medium red potatoes
2 red bell peppers, each cut lengthwise into eighths
8 small zucchini, trimmed and halved crosswise

1. Preheat oven to 350°. Cut 12 slits or pockets in top of lamb with tip of a small knife and fill each with ½ garlic clove. Place lamb on a rack in a large roasting pan.

2. Brush 3 or 4 tablespoons red pepper jelly over top of lamb. Insert meat thermometer into thickest part of lamb, being careful not to touch bone or fat. Surround lamb with potatoes. Roast, uncovered, 1 hour.

3. Remove lamb from oven and place 6 red pepper pieces on top of lamb and remainder around sides of lamb in pan. Add zucchini to roasting pan. Return to oven and continue roasting 1 to 1¼ hours longer, or until lamb is done to desired degree of doneness. Roast to 140° on thermometer for rare, 150–155° for medium, or 160° for medium-well.

4. Let lamb stand for 10 to 15 minutes for easier slicing. Serve lamb slices with potatoes, peppers, and zucchini. Pass remaining pepper jelly on the side.

---

349   SWEET POTATO AND APPLE STUFFED DUCK
Prep: 20 minutes   Cook: 1¾ hours   Serves: 3

This special roast duck would make a lovely holiday offering. Surround with plenty of watercress or other greens for a festive centerpiece. Since duck is very fatty, it doesn't go far. One duck serves three, at the most four. Initially roast the bird at a high temperature to ensure a crisp, beautiful, juicy bird. Keep in mind that the stuffing mixture used here would also be good in roasted chicken or Cornish game hens.

1 (5-pound) duckling, thawed if frozen
   Salt and pepper
1 (29-ounce) can cut yams, drained and cut into bite-size chunks
1 large tart green apple, chopped
½ cup chopped onion
2 tablespoons brown sugar

⅓ cup chopped pecans
¼ cup frozen orange juice concentrate, thawed
1 pound baby zucchini and baby crookneck yellow squash (or use cut-up chunks of regular zucchini and yellow squash)

1. Preheat oven to 450°. Remove neck, liver, and giblets from inside duckling. Trim off and discard any fat. Rinse and drain duckling. Pat dry with paper towels inside and out. Season inside with salt and pepper.

2. For stuffing, mix together yams, apple, onion, brown sugar, pecans, and 3 tablespoons undiluted orange juice concentrate.

3. Loosely fill neck and body cavities with stuffing. (Wrap any extra stuffing in a double thickness of foil and bake in oven along with duck the last ½ hour of roasting time.) Skewer neck and body cavity to close. Place duck, breast side up, on a rack in a shallow foil-lined roasting pan. Add ¼ cup water to pan to prevent spattering. Prick duck skin all over with a fork, without puncturing meat. Brush remaining 1 tablespoon orange juice concentrate over duck skin. Season with salt and pepper.

4. Roast duck 20 to 25 minutes. Reduce oven temperature to 350° and continue roasting 1¼ to 1½ hours longer, or until duck is tender and juices run clear. Last 45 minutes of roasting time, place squash on rack surrounding duck. Remove stuffing from duck cavities and serve with sliced duck and squash.

350 OVEN-BARBECUED RIBS WITH VEGETABLE PACKETS
Prep: 10 minutes   Cook: 1 to 1¼ hours   Serves: 4

If you love beef ribs, these are delicious and hassle-free. Bake foil packets of vegetables alongside and you have an oven-barbecued meal with little effort.

1　cup thick hickory-flavored barbecue sauce
2　tablespoons Dijon mustard
4　to 4½ pounds beef barbecue ribs
2　ears fresh corn, husked and halved
½　bunch broccoli, separated into florets (2 cups)

1　red bell pepper, quartered and each quarter cut into 6 pieces
4　large red or medium baking potatoes, thinly sliced
4　teaspoons butter
2　teaspoons minced fresh dill or 1 teaspoon dried
　　Salt and pepper

1. Preheat oven to 400°. Mix together barbecue sauce and mustard.

2. Place ribs on a foil-lined 10x15-inch jelly-roll pan. Brush with sauce mixture. Bake ribs 15 minutes.

3. Meanwhile prepare 4 individual foil packets (using a double thickness of foil, each sheet about 12x16 inches), dividing corn, broccoli, red pepper, and potato slices evenly among them. Dot each with 1 teaspoon butter and a sprinkling of dill. Season with salt and pepper. Wrap securely and pinch the edges to seal.

4. Place vegetable packets on oven rack around pan of ribs. Bake 15 minutes. Baste ribs with remaining sauce mixture and bake 30 to 45 minutes longer, until ribs are tender and browned and corn and potatoes are tender. Serve ribs with vegetables from packets.

351 SMOKED TURKEY AND ROASTED PEPPER PIZZA
Prep: 10 minutes   Cook: 15 to 18 minutes   Serves: 6

My daughter thinks this tastes like a chic California restaurant creation— she loves it.

1　pound prepared pizza dough (purchase at an Italian deli or market or use homemade) or frozen white bread dough, thawed
1　tablespoon olive oil
1½　cups shredded mozzarella cheese (6 ounces)

½　cup chopped roasted red peppers (a 7-ounce jar)
2　tablespoons chopped fresh basil
1　cup chopped smoked cooked turkey breast
2　scallions, chopped
¼　pound fresh mushrooms, sliced

1. Preheat oven to 500° if using pizza dough or 475° if using bread dough.

Roll out dough (using rolling pin and floured pastry cloth) or stretch pizza dough to fit into a 12-inch pizza pan.

2. Spread or brush olive oil over dough. Sprinkle evenly with cheese, red pepper, basil, turkey, scallions, and mushrooms.

3. Bake 15 to 18 minutes, or until crust is golden and pizza is cooked through.

352 SMOKED TURKEY BURRITO PIZZA
Prep: 10 minutes   Cook: 12 to 15 minutes   Serves: 4

The flavors of a burrito are rolled into this novel pizza, which is a wonderful meal-in-a-dish. Top with a dollop of sour cream and sprinkle with chopped fresh tomatoes and shredded lettuce, if desired.

1 **(1-pound) loaf frozen white bread dough, thawed, or 1 pound prepared pizza dough (homemade or purchased at an Italian market)**
1 **(16-ounce) can refried beans with green chiles**
⅓ **cup mild thick and chunky salsa**
2 **scallions, chopped**

2 **tablespoons chopped fresh cilantro (optional)**
1 **cup chopped smoked turkey breast or chicken**
2 **cups shredded cheddar cheese (8 ounces)**
Sour cream, chopped tomatoes, and shredded lettuce, as accompaniment

1. Preheat oven to 450° (500° if using pizza dough).

2. Roll (using a rolling pin and floured pastry cloth) or stretch dough to fit into a lightly greased 12-inch pizza pan, building up edges slightly.

3. Mix beans with salsa and spread over top of dough, leaving ½-inch border around the edges. Sprinkle scallions, cilantro, turkey, and cheese evenly over pizza.

4. Bake in middle of oven 12 to 15 minutes, or until crust is golden. Cut into 8 to 10 wedges to serve. Pass sour cream, chopped tomato, and shredded lettuce on the side.

353   BARBECUED CHICKEN PIZZA

Prep: 10 minutes   Cook: 12 to 15 minutes   Serves: 4

Here's a trendy pizza that has been popularized in California and now
has traveled throughout the country.

1 pound prepared pizza
  dough (purchased at an
  Italian market or
  homemade)
1 cup barbecue sauce
3 thin slices red onion, halved
  and separated into pieces

2 cups chopped barbecued
  chicken
3 cups shredded smoked
  Gouda or mozzarella
  cheese
3 tablespoons chopped fresh
  basil or cilantro

1. Preheat oven to 500°. Roll out or stretch pizza dough to fit into a lightly
greased 12-inch pizza pan.

2. Spread barbecue sauce evenly over dough just to the edges. Sprinkle
evenly with red onion pieces, chicken, cheese, and basil.

3. Bake on top shelf of oven 12 to 15 minutes, or until crust is golden. Cut
into 8 to 10 wedges to serve.

354   HAMBURGER PIZZA

Prep: 15 minutes   Cook: 35 minutes   Serves: 5 to 6

Be sure to use the leanest beef possible for this one-dish meal reminiscent
of a meat loaf but with a pizza-like topping. This is a favorite of children and
adults alike. Vary the toppings—add sliced mushrooms, sliced ripe olives,
chopped green pepper, and more.

2 pounds lean ground round
1 (10-ounce) package frozen
  chopped spinach, thawed
  (do not drain)
2 slices whole wheat bread
  with crust on, torn into
  cubes
1 egg
½ cup milk
½ teaspoon pepper
1 tablespoon Worcestershire
  sauce

1 medium onion, chopped
1 cup quick-cooking long-
  grain rice
1 (8-ounce) can tomato sauce
1 teaspoon Italian seasoning
1 teaspoon basil
1 garlic clove, minced
3 ounces thinly sliced salami
  or pepperoni
1 cup shredded mozzarella
  cheese (4 ounces)

1. Preheat oven to 425°. Combine beef, undrained spinach, bread cubes,
egg, milk, pepper, Worcestershire sauce, onion, and rice. Mix to blend well.
Turn into a 12-inch pizza pan with a ¾-inch-high edge; do not use a flat
pizza pan. Bake 25 minutes. Remove from oven. Drain off any fat.

2. Blend tomato sauce with Italian seasoning, basil, and garlic. Spread over
pizza. Top with slices of salami. Sprinkle with cheese. Return to oven and
continue baking 10 minutes. Cut into wedges to serve.

355 PESTO-SHRIMP PIZZA
Prep: 15 minutes   Cook: 12 to 15 minutes   Serves: 3 to 4

For an upscale pizza, try this version without tomato sauce and cheese. Pesto sauce, either store-bought or homemade, goes atop the crust before topping with shrimp, tomatoes (fresh and sun-dried), and olives. Serve with a large bowl of tossed greens to complete the meal.

5 to 6 tablespoons pesto sauce
1 (12-inch) unbaked pizza crust (use pizza dough or frozen bread dough, thawed and rolled out to fit into pizza pan)
1 large fresh tomato, seeded and chopped

2 tablespoons chopped sun-dried tomatoes packed in oil
⅓ cup coarsely chopped ripe olives
1 cup peeled and deveined frozen shrimp, thawed and well drained

1. Preheat oven to 475°. Spread pesto sauce over unbaked pizza crust. Sprinkle top evenly with fresh and sun-dried tomatoes, then olives and shrimp.

2. Bake 12 to 15 minutes, or until golden. Cut into 8 to 10 wedges.

356 TORTILLA VEGETABLE PIZZA
Prep: 10 minutes   Cook: 12 to 15 minutes   Serves: 4

Flour tortillas make a great base for individual dinner pizzas. And they bake in a jiffy, too. Alter the topping ingredients to suit personal tastes.

4 (7½-inch) flour tortillas
1 cup shredded carrots (2 large carrots)
1 cup shredded zucchini
1 cup sliced fresh mushrooms
1 (2.2-ounce) can sliced ripe olives, drained
2 scallions, chopped

1 cup chopped hickory-smoked cooked turkey or chicken
1 (7-ounce) can green chile salsa
1½ cups shredded cheddar or Monterey Jack cheese

1. Preheat oven to 375°. Place tortillas flat on 2 large baking sheets. Bake 4 to 5 minutes to crisp.

2. In a medium bowl, combine carrots, zucchini, mushrooms, olives, scallions, and turkey. Mix well.

3. Spread 2 tablespoons salsa on each tortilla. Sprinkle each tortilla with turkey mixture. Top each with cheese and drizzle each with some of remaining salsa.

4. Bake 8 to 10 minutes, until cheese has melted and vegetables are hot. Serve 1 per person, each cut into 4 wedges.

357   QUICK PITA PIZZAS
Prep: 10 minutes   Cook: 5 to 8 minutes   Serves: 4

When there's no time to think about a quick dinner or lunch, whip up these quick pizzas in a jiffy. Sprinkle the cheese with assorted cooked vegetables or meats, depending on what's handy in the refrigerator. Accompany with a tossed green salad, and a meal is on the table in short order.

2 (9- or 10-inch) pita breads
1 cup pizza sauce
2 cups shredded cheddar and mozzarella cheeses
1 (2.2-ounce) can sliced ripe olives, drained

¾ cup chopped leftover cooked vegetables (broccoli, zucchini, eggplant, and/or peppers)
1 cup chopped cooked meat (ham, turkey, chicken, salami, and/or sausage)

1. Preheat oven to 450°. Split each pita bread into 2 thin rounds. Arrange cut sides up on baking sheets. Spread each with about 3 generous tablespoons pizza sauce and sprinkle each with ½ cup cheese. Top with a sprinkling of olives, vegetables, and meat.

2. Bake 5 to 8 minutes, until pizza is very hot and cheese is melted. With a sharp knife, cut into wedges to serve.

358   FAST SOUTHWESTERN PIZZA
Prep: 5 minutes   Cook: 8 to 10 minutes   Serves: 4

Take the easy way out and prepare this pizza with Boboli—a ready-made, prebaked cheese crust—as the base. Vary the toppings to suit what you have on hand in the refrigerator and on your pantry shelf.

1 (16-ounce) package prebaked refrigerated 12-inch diameter cheese crust (Boboli)
½ cup mild or hot green chile salsa
1 (7-ounce) can Mexicorn (whole kernel corn with red and green peppers), drained

¾ cup chopped boiled or baked sliced ham (3 ounces)
1 cup shredded Monterey Jack cheese (4 ounces)
1 (2.2-ounce) can sliced ripe olives, rinsed and drained

1. Preheat oven to 500°. Place crust on baking sheet. Spread salsa evenly over crust. Sprinkle half the corn and half the ham over salsa, then sprinkle cheese evenly over all. Top with remaining corn and ham and the olives.

2. Bake 8 to 10 minutes, until crust is golden and cheese is melted. Cut into wedges to serve.

359   MEAT AND SPINACH TORTE
Prep: 20 minutes   Cook: 50 minutes   Serves: 10

This torte creation combines meats, cheese, and spinach in a rich puff pastry crust. It's a fabulous choice for a special brunch, luncheon, or sophisticated picnic. Although it may appear complicated to make, it's really simple once all the ingredients are assembled.

1 (17 ¼-ounce) package frozen puff pastry
⅓ cup grated Parmesan cheese
1 (6-ounce) package Monterey Jack or Swiss cheese slices
¾ pound thinly sliced cooked ham
¼ pound salami slices
3 (10-ounce) packages frozen chopped spinach, thawed and squeezed dry

1 (16-ounce) container ricotta cheese
2 eggs
2 scallions, chopped
½ teaspoon garlic powder
½ teaspoon salt
¼ teaspoon pepper
1 (7-ounce) jar roasted red peppers, drained

1. Thaw pastry sheets 30 to 45 minutes and unfold. On a lightly floured surface, roll out one pastry sheet to a large circle that measures about 17 inches in diameter. Ease pastry into a 10-inch springform pan and gently press against bottom and sides, leaving a ½-inch overhang.

2. Preheat oven to 425°. To assemble torte, sprinkle 2 tablespoons Parmesan cheese over bottom of prepared pastry. Top with layers of half the Jack cheese slices, half the ham slices, and half the salami slices.

3. Mix together spinach, ricotta cheese, 1 egg, scallions, garlic powder, salt, and pepper. Spread spinach mixture evenly over salami layer. Top with all roasted peppers, opened flat. Top with remaining salami, followed by remaining ham and Jack cheese slices. Sprinkle with remaining Parmesan cheese.

4. Roll remaining pastry sheet on a lightly floured surface into an 11-inch circle. Ease crust over filling in springform. Fold up edges of top crust and roll overhanging crust inward to seal, pinching to form a decorative border, if desired.

5. Beat remaining egg and brush over entire top of torte. With a sharp thin knife, make several small cuts in top pastry to allow for steam to escape. Set pan on a piece of foil and wrap sides of foil up around pan to catch any leakage that may occur during baking.

6. Bake 10 minutes, then reduce oven temperature to 400° and continue baking 40 minutes longer, or until top is golden brown. Cool on wire rack at least 30 minutes before removing springform side. Serve torte warm or at room temperature. Keep any leftovers refrigerated.

360   GUACAMOLE-BRIE SANDWICH
Prep: 10 minutes   Cook: 5 to 8 minutes   Serves: 4

This unlikely combination is sensational sandwich fare for lunch or supper accompanied with a tossed green or fruit salad.

1 (8-ounce) sourdough or French bread
1 large ripe avocado
2 tablespoons lemon juice
¼ teaspoon garlic salt
⅛ teaspoon pepper
1 tablespoon bottled Italian herb dressing
2 to 3 tablespoons minced fresh basil

5 to 6 ounces cold Brie, rind removed, cheese thinly sliced
¼ cup finely chopped oil-packed sun-dried tomatoes, drained (6 to 8 dried tomatoes)

1. Preheat oven to 350°. Split bread in half lengthwise with a sharp knife. Place, cut sides up, on a foil-lined baking sheet.

2. Make a guacamole by mashing avocado with lemon juice, garlic salt, and pepper. Spread guacamole on bread, dividing evenly between the 2 halves.

3. Sprinkle with Italian dressing; spread out with a knife. Sprinkle basil over guacamole. Arrange Brie slices on top. Sprinkle sun-dried tomatoes over cheese.

4. Bake 5 to 8 minutes, or until cheese is melted.

361   GREEK-STYLE SPINACH PIE
Prep: 30 minutes   Cook: 45 minutes   Serves: 10 to 12

Don't be intimidated by filo dough, but keep in mind you must work quickly when using it. There's no need to worry about tears or mistakes either, as they won't show in the finished dish. This creation can be used for an entrée as well as hors d'oeuvre, depending on the size the pieces are cut.

3 (10-ounce) packages frozen chopped spinach, thawed and squeezed dry
2 cups (16 ounces) low-fat cottage cheese
8 ounces feta cheese, crumbled (2 cups)
1 small onion or 5 scallions, finely chopped

4 eggs
1½ teaspoons dried dill weed
1 (1-pound) package filo dough sheets (thaw in refrigerator if purchased frozen)
1 stick plus 2 tablespoons butter, melted

1. Preheat oven to 350°. In a medium bowl, combine spinach, cottage cheese, feta cheese, onion, eggs, and dill weed. Mix to blend well.

2. Open and stack filo sheets on a damp towel. Trim long side of stack of sheets to fit into a 10x15-inch jelly-roll pan. Butter pan.

3. Layer 8 filo sheets in buttered pan, brushing each sheet with melted butter. Then drape 2 sheets of buttered phyllo over the long sides of the pan, one on each side.

4. Spread spinach mixture evenly over entire pan of filo. Fold draped side pieces of filo over filling. Brush filo with butter. Top with remaining filo sheets, brushing each with butter. Turn edges under. Brush top with remaining butter.

5. Bake about 45 minutes, or until golden. Let stand 5 to 10 minutes. Cut into squares and serve warm for a supper, brunch, or luncheon entrée.

> **NOTE:** *This freezes and reheats well in a conventional oven.*

---

362 SUNDAY FOOTBALL SANDWICH SENSATION
Prep: 15 to 20 minutes   Cook: none   Serves: 6 to 8

Absolutely delicious and fabulous looking. A conversation piece!

1 (1½-pound) round loaf unsliced Italian or French bread
1 (6-ounce) jar sweet fried peppers with onions, drained
1 (4¼-ounce) can chopped ripe olives, drained
1 small red onion, chopped
½ head iceberg lettuce, shredded (about 4 cups)
½ cup bottled Italian dressing

1½ pounds thinly sliced deli meats (mortadella, salami, and pepperoni)
1 pound thinly sliced deli cheeses (mozzarella and provolone)
2 large tomatoes, sliced ¼-inch thick
Baby carrots, radishes, scallions, pickled hot peppers (pepperoncini), and ripe olives, for accompaniments

1. Split bread horizontally through center.

2. In a large bowl, combine peppers and onions, chopped olives, red onion, and lettuce. Add dressing and toss to coat salad.

3. Place half the salad mixture on bottom half of bread. Top with layers of assorted meats, cheeses, tomatoes, meats, and cheeses. Top with remaining lettuce mixture and repeat layers of meats, cheese, and tomatoes. Cover with top half of bread, pressing down firmly. Loaf will be piled high. Cut into wedges to serve. Accompany with carrots, radishes, scallions, pepperoncini, and olives.

> **NOTE:** *Loaf can be prepared 2 to 3 hours in advance of serving. Wrap well and keep refrigerated.*

363   CHEESE AND HAM–STUFFED LOAF
Prep: 15 minutes   Cook: 30 to 35 minutes   Serves: 6

This is not only easy to make, but fun to serve. Hollow out a long loaf of Italian or French bread, fill with a tasty ham and cheese mixture, and bake until heated through. Refrigerate any leftovers and eat cold. Keep this in mind for picnic fare, too.

1 **large loaf Italian or French bread (about 15 inches long and 4½ inches wide)**
1 **(3-ounce) package cream cheese, softened**
½ **cup sour cream**
1 **(10-ounce) package frozen chopped spinach, thawed and squeezed dry**

3 **scallions, chopped**
¼ **cup chopped red bell pepper**
2 **cups shredded cheddar cheese (8 ounces)**
½ **pound cooked ham, chopped**

1. Preheat oven to 375°. Slice off top of loaf; set aside. Pull out soft inside of loaf (reserve for another use), leaving a thick shell.

2. Mix together cream cheese and sour cream until smooth. Stir in spinach, scallions, red pepper, cheddar cheese, and ham; blend well. Spoon into hollowed-out loaf. Replace top of loaf.

3. Wrap loaf tightly in heavy-duty aluminum foil. Bake 30 to 35 minutes, or until heated through. To serve, cut into diagonal slices.

364   BAKED BRUNCH OMELETS
Prep: 10 minutes   Cook: 18 to 20 minutes   Serves: 6

If you want something easy and festive to serve guests at brunch, these individual omelets are worthy of consideration. Have them ready to pop into the oven shortly after guests arrive. This is also a nice idea for a simple supper. You can substitute leftover cooked ham for the bacon, if desired.

12 **thin slices Canadian bacon or cooked ham, diced**
8 **eggs**
½ **cup sour cream**
1 **(6-ounce) can pitted ripe olives, drained and cut into pieces**

2 **scallions, chopped**
⅓ **cup chopped red bell pepper**
1 **cup shredded Swiss, Monterey Jack, or cheddar cheese (4 ounces)**

1. Preheat oven to 350°. Line bottom of 6 individual gratin dishes or ramekins (5½x1-inch) with cut-up bacon, dividing evenly.

2. With a whisk, beat eggs with sour cream until well blended. Stir in olives, scallions, red pepper, and cheese.

3. Pour mixture over bacon in 6 prepared dishes, dividing evenly. Bake 18 to 20 minutes, or until eggs are set (baking time will depend on depth of mixture in dishes).

365   BAKED HAM AND CHEESEWICH
Prep: 15 minutes   Cook: 20 to 25 minutes   Serves: 4

Stuff a spinach, ham, and cheese filling in a loaf of frozen bread for a meal. It's almost as easy as making a sandwich. A simple salad or bowl of vegetable soup is all you need to complete the menu.

1 (1-pound) loaf frozen white bread dough, thawed
1 to 2 tablespoons prepared yellow mustard
¼ pound cooked ham slices
1 (6-ounce) package Swiss or Monterey Jack cheese slices

5 ounces fresh spinach, stemmed, washed, and dried
1 egg white, beaten

1. Lightly flour a pastry cloth or a piece of wax paper. Place bread dough on cloth; sprinkle dough lightly with flour. With a rolling pin, roll out dough to a 10x14-inch rectangle.

2. Spread mustard lengthwise down center third of dough. Top with ham, then cheese and spinach. Make cuts in dough from filling to dough edges at 1-inch intervals along sides of filling. Alternating sides, fold cut strips at a slight angle over top of filling to cover.

3. Carefully transfer filled dough loaf to a greased baking sheet. Let rise in a warm place 15 to 20 minutes.

4. Meanwhile, preheat oven to 375°. Brush top of loaf with egg white. Bake 20 to 25 minutes, or until golden brown. Serve warm, cut into slices. Refrigerate any leftovers.

Index

About the Author

Natalie Haughton graduated from the University of California at Davis with a degree in home economics. Her talents for writing, recipe development, and food styling for photography have been honed at jobs in advertising and public relations as well as with major food companies and consumer education organizations.

Food editor at the Los Angeles Daily News since 1976, Haughton has been a chocophile since birth. She is the author of *Cookies* (HP Books) and resides with her husband and two children in Studio City, California.